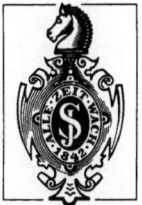

P. C. Braga L. Allegra (Eds.)

Lungscapes

With 94 Color Figures

Springer-Verlag
Berlin Heidelberg New York
London Paris Tokyo
Hong Kong Barcelona
Budapest

Pier Carlo Braga, M.D.
Centro di Farmacologia Respiratoria
Via Vanvitelli, 32
I-20129 Milano, Italy

Luigi Allegra, M.D.
Istituto di Malattie Respiratorie
Policlinico – Pad. Litta
Via F. Sforza, 35
I-20100 Milano, Italy

ISBN 978-88-470-2257-7   ISBN 978-88-470-2255-3 (eBook)
DOI   10.1007/978-88-470-2255-3

Typesetting: Elsner & Behrens GmbH, Oftersheim, FRG

25/3145/PE-543210 – Printed on acid-free paper

"God Bless the Microscope
… and Microscopists too"

"One Picture is Worth
more than a Thousand Words"

Preface

The invention of an instrument called the optical microscope and the new possibilities it offered to observe living material must be considered a major milestone in the advance of our understanding of the mechanisms of life. Huge numbers of important observations have been made using this instrument, but unfortunately it only produces two-dimensional images. The advent of the electron microscope, first the transmission electron microscope (TEM) and then the scanning electron microscope (SEM), then made it possible to observe the three-dimensional structure of specimens literally adding a whole new dimension to our understanding and bringing about a second major milestone in microscopy.

With their highly specific architecture and great functional significance, the respiratory apparatus and the airways have received particular attention, and extensive series of investigations with SEM have been done. "To see is to understand", and many lung SEM investigations with different aims have been performed, but "to see again is to understand better", so we offer this collection of scanning electron micrographs, which, along with some familiar aspects, also presents new and unusual images of pulmonary morphology.

We have noticed that although most pulmonary structures have already been seen, every time we scan a new specimen, new perspectives, new aspects, and new details emerge. We hope that physicians and scientists looking at these scanning electron micrographs will, just as we did, find new sources of wonder, and will then desire to delve deeper.

This collection of images is addressed not just to pneumologists, but to all physicians, and so we have selected images taken using SEM, which are more readily understood than TEM images. In addition, images relating to different topics have different colors to aid in identifying and differentiating the specific topographical aspects of the lung.

Milano, March 1992

Pier Carlo Braga
Luigi Allegra

Acknowledgements

Taking of human biological samples, technical preparation of the specimens, setting and running the scanning electron microscope, preparing the micrographs, and discussing the findings is a complex task that generally involves more than one person. We are therefore grateful to Prof. P. Belloni and all his staff (Thoracic Surgery Division, Niguarda Hospital, Milan) who gave us pulmonary tissue samples from different surgical situations. We also wish to express our appreciation to Prof. F. Clementi (Department of Pharmacology, School of Medicine, University of Milan) for use of the microscope and related apparatus, to Prof. C. De Giuli Morghen (Department of Pharmacology, School of Medicine, University of Milan) for his help and suggestions, and to Prof. P. Castano (Institute of Anatomy, School of Pharmacy, University of Milan) for providing us with some scanning electron micrographs from his collection. We are especially indebted to Dr. G. Piatti (grant recipient from the Center for Respiratory Pharmacology), who worked extensively with us in preparing this collection of micrographs, for her tireless efforts. Finally, special thanks are due to Dompè Farmaceutici for its support and constant help.

Contents

Chapter 1
Scanning Electron Microscopy: Notes on Basic Techniques for Investigating Pulmonary and Airway Structures

P. C. Braga

Centro di Farmacologia Respiratoria, Facoltà di Medicina e Chirurgia,
Università degli Studi di Milano

Introduction

The eye is probably the most important "sensor" of our body. Not only does it provide information about our surroundings, but this information is then used by the brain to control our interaction with the surroundings through feedback. It is a common observation that we cannot see structural details of either very minute objects or of larger objects at great distance, so the idea of magnifying images of the things that surround us has always fascinated man. From the earliest times, discoveries of magnifying devices such as drops of water, convex metal mirrors, and lenses have been reported, with records dating back to 1000 B.C. or even earlier. The Assyrians had a convex lens around 700 B.C., and the Greeks and Romans also wrote about magnifying lenses [1].

The production of an instrument called the "microscope" between the end of the sixteenth century and the beginning of the seventeenth century was then, a true breakthrough in the advance of civilization [2]. The microscope is a device which utilizes a combination of lenses to obtain magnifications never before attained, thus making it possible to observe the "microcosmos" of the minute details of materials and of living organisms that had never been suspected to exist before.

The continuous improvement of this instrument and its use in observing nature around us and the human body are very important contributions to human knowledge in general and to the present body of medical knowledge: without the microscope, natural, biological, and medical sciences would not be what they are today.

The optical microscope can be used for many kinds of observaton, but it has a limit in its capacity to resolve structures. The naked eye, for instance, cannot separate two dots printed less than 0.1 millimiters apart [3], while the resolution of the optical microscope is about 0.001 mm, that is to say, it enlarges by 1000 times. With special equipment and techniques, this enlargement can be increased, but still the wavelength of visible light imposes a definite limit on optical resolving power.

After the optical microscope, a second breakthrough serving to satisfy man's impulse to expand his consciousness was the development of the electron microscope, which now has a history of about 50 years [4]. The electron microscope, using electrons with wavelengths of much less than 0.1 nm ($= 1\text{Å}$ or ångström $= 1 \times 10^{-10}$ m or one ten-billionth of a meter) greatly increased resolving power, along with depth of field and depth of focus: high magnification is of little use if not accompanied by high resolution.

Electron microscopes can be divided into two major types: transmission electron microscopes (TEMs), the first developed, explore the internal structure of a thin specimen two-dimensionally, while scanning electron microscopes (SEMs) provide three-dimensional images of the surface morphology of specimens [5].

The Basic Elements of the SEM

The function of the scanning electron microscopy (SEM) is basically similar to that of an optical microscope, but instead of light it uses an electron

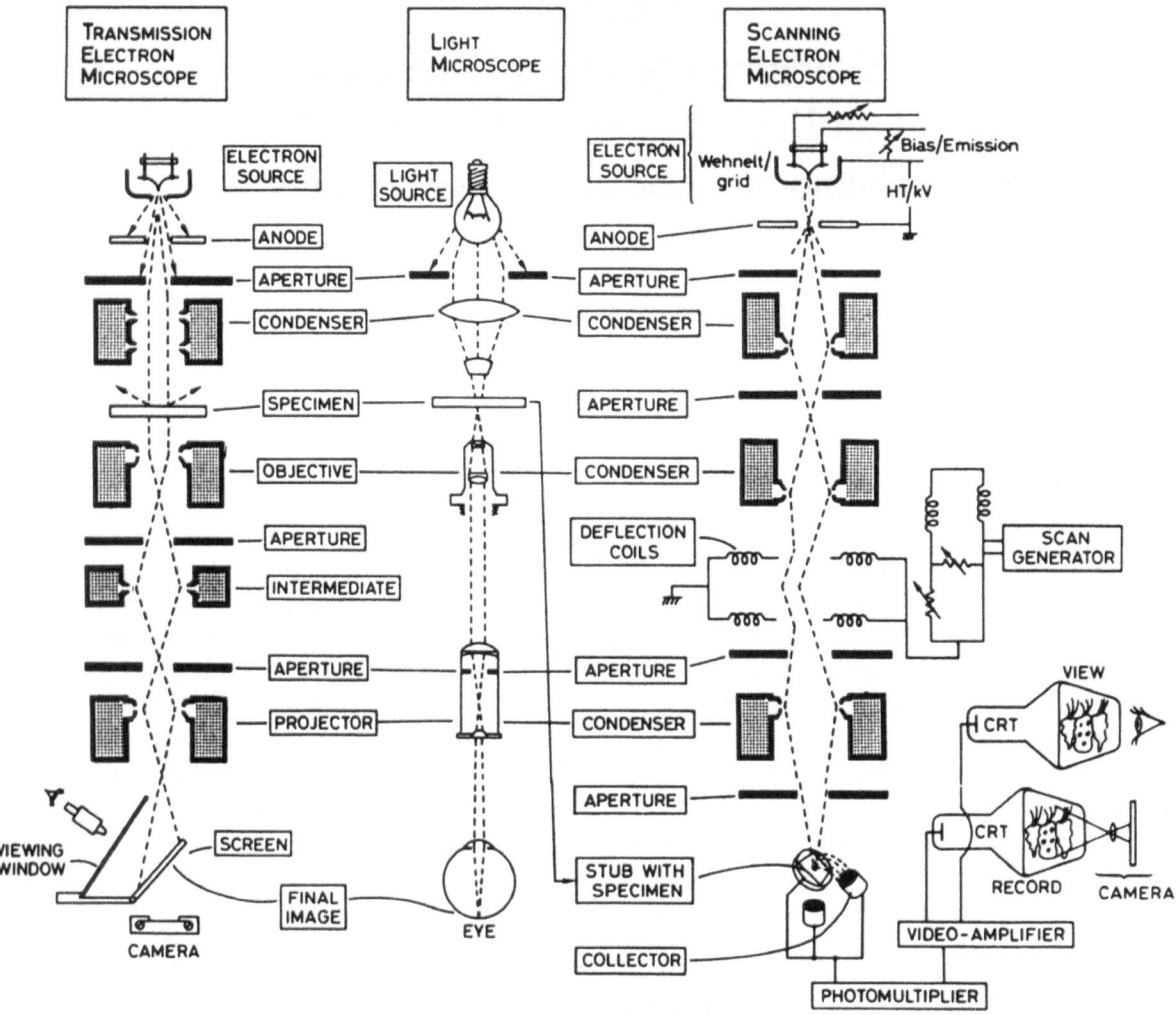

Fig. 1.1. Schematic diagram of the elements characterizing light microscopes, transmission electron microscopes, and scanning electron microscopes

beam to explore the specimen, and instead of a lens of glass it uses magnetic coils as a lens (electromagnetic lens) to drive electrons (Fig. 1.1).

The Source of Electrons

A "pointed tungsten filament" (diameter 0.1 mm) is the most common source of electrons. When a suitable current flows through this filament, it is heated to a high temperature (white heat, 2500–2600 K) and releases many thermoionic electrons. These are accelerated towards an anode and pass through a hole in the grid so that at the end an

electron beam is generated. This part of the system is also called the "thermoionic electron gun."

The Vacuum System

To minimize the scattering of the electron beam by air molecules (collision of electrons with air molecules makes a very "noisy" signal) and permit the electrons to reach the specimen, it is essential to remove most of the air from the column of the microscope using a vacuum system. A second important function of the vacuum is to prevent the specimen, the apertures, or the electron gun from becoming contaminated by material entering the column and being depositing on them. Different combinations of rotatory, turbomolecular, diffusion, ion, and cryogenic pumps are used to obtain the vacuum, which for the SEM is generally between 10^{-3} and 10^{-6} Torr.

The Electromagnetic Lenses

Basically, an electromagnetic lens is a coil of many turns of wire bound around a hollow cylinder (a solenoid). Such a solenoid has a magnetic field along its axis and acts as an adjustable lens on an electron beam passing through it, because the strength of the magnetic field and, hence, the focal length of the lens can be varied by altering the current in the coil, thus changing the magnifying power of the lens [6]. In the column of the SEM there are condenser lenses, stigmator lenses; like glass lenses, magnetic lenses have chromatic, spherical, and astigmatic aberrations that must be corrected for.

The Detection System

The stub bearing the specimen can be moved along three axes *(x, y, z)* and tilted and rotated. In the specimen chamber, the tiny beam of electrons strikes the specimen and interacts with its surface, generating other electrons with different energies that then radiate outwards. These "secondary electrons" are collected by a detector (scintillator plus photomultiplier tube), the output current of which is amplified and transmitted to a cathode ray tube (television monitor).

The presence of a "scan generator" enables the electron beam (diameter 100–300 nm) to scan the specimen in a series of lines and frames, called "raster scan", so that, finally, a series of spots of light of different intensities are produced on the television screen to form a complete amplified image of the specimen's surface that can be photographed [7]. For routine viewing, a long-persistence phosphorescent screen is adopted, while for taking pictures a high-resolution, short-persistence phosphorescent screen is used.

While TEM gives magnifications of up to 1000000 times, SEM can provide a range of magnifications from about 15 to 200000 times, depending on the nature and form of the material examined. Higher magnifications can be obtained with more sophisticated instruments. The resolving power of a light microscope is about 2500 Å, while for SEM a resolution of 100 Å at 30 kV is common.

A light microscope allows one to examine both nonliving and living material, while TEM and SEM require samples to be dry and examined in a vacuum, so only nonliving materials can be observed. Living material must undergo specific processing before SEM.

SEM has many advantages and provides kinds of information not provided by TEM or light microscopy. These advantages include [8], for instance, a very great depth of field, resulting in three-dimensional images; the ability to view a larger specimen than in TEM and light microscopy; a broad range of magnifications; high resolution; and ease of varying the magnification without changing the focal length, so that the depth of the field remains constant.

SEM Techniques

As already mentioned, the internal environment of SEM is under vacuum, so fresh biological soft tissue or living material cannot be observed because the water within the cell and in the extracellular space would vaporize explosively when exposed to the vacuum of 10^{-3}–10^{-6} Torr [9]. Moreover, the surface tension forces generated during evaporation and the resulting formation and growth of ice crystals would render the resulting images almost worthless [8]. Therefore, depending on the nature of sample, different preparation techniques are adopted to preserve the natural morphology as well as possible.

Chemical Fixation

After careful collection and manipulation of biological samples to avoid stretching or touching the tissue surface, the specimens must be fixed to quickly stabilize all the molecular and macromolecular components of cell and tissue architecture. This is done, within certain limitations, by using chemical fixatives. A wide variety of these compounds have been employed for SEM study of biological tissues [10–12]. Commonly employed fixatives are osmium tetroxide [13, 14], glutaraldehyde [15, 16], Karnovsky's fixative [17], and mixtures of the above and other compounds [18]. The pH of these solutions must be between 6.5 and 8.0, and several kinds of buffer can be used to keep the pH between 7.2 and 7.4. Hypertonicity or hypotonicity can cause shrinkage or swelling of cells, so osmolarity must also be controlled [19–21]. Different time schedules of fixation and temperature are used according to the size and kind of specimen.

Dehydration

This step in the procedure is (performed) to remove water and other fluids from the specimen to avoid the shrinkage phenomena and deformation that occur if fixed tissues are dried without previous dehydration. One common dehydration procedure is to pass the specimen through graded series of either ethanol or acetone (e.g., 30%, 50%, 70%, 85%, 95%, 100%) for different times [8].

Critical Point Drying

When a tissue is air dried, large surface tension forces arise in zones of contact between liquid and gas, and distortion occurs. The most common drying procedure at present is the "critical point method", using liquid carbon dioxide [22]. This technique, introduced by Anderson [22], involves various steps, namely alcohol substitution with liquid CO_2, heating to super critical temperature for CO_2 sublimation, and then pressure release. This technique is based on the fact that at its critical point liquid CO_2 passes imperceptibly from a liquid to a gas with no evident boundary and no associated distortional force [8]. In any case, a certain degree of shrinkage of soft tissues will occur [23–26]. A number of commercially available devices for critical point drying are on the market.

Mounting and Metal Coating

After the above-mentioned steps, the specimen is attached with a thin layer of silver-based conducting paint to the stub, which is made of brass or aluminum. The stubs vary in shape depending on the type of SEM. The stub with specimen is then transferred to a vacuum evaporator, where the specimen is coated by a sputtering method with a thin layer of gold (5–30 nm) to increase its electrical conductance [27–30].

Supplementary Techniques

Many other different techniques or modifications of the techniques described above are in use for SEM observations [31–35]. One interesting technique which is complementary to those that permit the observation of surfaces of cells and tissues is the "cryofracture" or freeze-fracture technique, with which one can observe both extracellular or intracellular surfaces of the specimen [36–39]. This new type of observation is obtained by freezing the specimen in liquid nitrogen or other medium [40] and then cracking it in a half with a razor blade [41].

Applications of SEM to Investigation of the Lung

Since 1966, when the SEM became commercially available, it has shown its great versatility in examining and analyzing the microstructural characteristics of biological specimens. The unusual topography of the respiratory system, with its channels conducting the air to the sponge-like alveolar structures, can be studied very well by SEM, which permits better observation of the structure of this particular organ than other kinds of investigations.

Initially, investigators employed air drying to prepare samples for SEM observation, and this resulted in shrinkage and distortion of the surface structure. The development by Anderson [22] of the critical point technique was the most significant turning point in the study of the lung by SEM.

In view of the peculiar structure of the alveolar part of the lung and its collapsibility, the commonly used fixation by immersion does not always preserve the original three-dimensional relationships between airways, vessels, and cells, so the inflation-fixation technique was adopted for better morphological preservation of the alveolar part of the lung. Rapid freezing, freeze-substitution techniques [42, 43], immunolabelling, and casting replicas of the alveoli and pulmonary vasculature are other techniques that have increased the number of ways the lung can be examined. As shown in later chapters of this atlas, SEM has aided in revealing the size, shape, architecture, density, and type of surface micro-projections characterizing the various respiratory cell types – ciliated, goblet, brush, Clara, alveolar, and nonresident cells (macrophages, etc.) – as well as the internal alveolar architecture, the relationships of these structures to each other and to bronchi and bronchioles [44] and mucus, surfactant, and pollutants, both in physiological and pathological conditions. As our introductory quotation says, "One picture is worth more than a thousand words": this appears particularly true for the respiratory system viewed by SEM.

References

1. Scharf D (1979) Magnifications, photography with the scanning electron microscope. Muller, London
2. Bradbury S (1968) The microscope, past and present. Pergamon, Oxford
3. Burgess J, Marten M, Taylor R (1987) Microcosmos. Cambridge University Press, Cambridge
4. McMullan D (1989) SEM, past, present and future. J Microsc 155:373–393
5. Chescoe D, Goodhew PJ (1990) The operation of transmission and scanning electron microscopes. Oxford University Press, Oxford
6. Watti M (1985) Principles and practice of electron microscopy. Cambridge University Press, Cambridge
7. Scala C, Pasquinelli G (1987) Microscopia elettronica a scansione in biologia. Editrice CLUEB, Bologna
8. Kessel RG, Shith CY (1976) Scanning electron microscopy in biology. Springer Berlin Heidelberg New York
9. Ross N, Morgan AJ (1990) Cryopreparation of thin biological specimens for electron microscopy: methods and applications. Oxford University Press, Oxford
10. Hayat (1981) Fixation for electron microscopy. Academic, New York
11. McDowell EM, Trump BF (1976) Histologic fixatives suitable for diagnostic light and electron microscopy. Arch Pathol Lab Med 100:405–414
12. Hulbert WC, Forster BB, Laird W, Phil CE, Walker DC (1982) An improved method for fixation of the respiratory epithelial surface with the mucous and surfactant layers. Lab Invest 47:354–363
13. Litman RB, Barrnett RJ (1982) The mechanism of the fixation of tissue components by osmium tetroxide via hydrogen binding J Ultrastr Res 38:63–86
14. Kelley RO, Dekker RAF, Bluemink JG (1973) Ligand-mediated osmium binding: its application in coating biological specimens for scanning electron microscopy. J Ultrastruct Res 45:254–258
15. Mathieu O, Claassen H, Weibel ER (1978) Differential effect of glutaraldehyde and buffer osmolarity on cell dimensions: a study on lung tissue. J Ultrastruct Res 63:20–34
16. Arborgh B, Bell P, Brunk U, Collins VP (1976) The osmotic effect of glutaraldehyde fixation. A transmission electron microscopy. Scanning electron microscopy and cytochemical study. J Ultrastruct Res 56:331–350
17. Karnovsky MJ (1965) A formaldeide-glutaraldehyde fixative of high osmolarity for use in electron microscopy. J Cell Biol 27:137–138 A
18. Katsumoto T, Naguro T, Iino A, Takagi A (1981) The effect of tannic acid on the preservation of tissue culture cells for scanning electron microscopy. J Electron Microsc (Tokyo) 30:177–182
19. Gil J, Weibel ER (1968) The role of buffers in lung fixation with glutaraldehyde and osmium tetroxide. J Ultrastruct Res 25:331–348
20. Schiff RI, Gennaro JF (1979) The role of the buffer in the fixation of biological specimens for transmission and scanning electron microscopy. Scanning 2:135–148
21. Boyde A (1976) Do's and don'ts in biological specimen preparation for the SEM. Scanning Electron Microsc 9:697–734
22. Anderson TF (1951) Techniques for the preservation of three-dimensional structure in preparing specimens for the electron microscope. Trans NY Acad Sci (Ser II) 13:130–134
23. Bastacky J, Hayes TL, Gelinas RP (1985) Quantitation of shrinkage during preparation for scanning electron microscopy: human lung. Scanning 7:134–140
24. Mazzone RW, Kornblau S, Durand CM (1980) Shrinkage of lung after chemical fixation for analysis of pulmonary structure-function relations. J Appl Physiol 48:382–385
25. Wollweber L, Stacke R, Gothe U (1981) The use of a simple methods to avoid cell shrinkage during SEM preparation. J Microsc 121:185–189

26. Inouè T, Osatake H (1988) A new drying method of biological specimens for scanning electron microscopy, the t-butyl-alcohol freeze-drying method. Arch Histol Cytol 51:53–59

27. Echlin P (1975) Sputter coating techniques for scanning electron microscopy. Scanning Electron Microsc 8:217–224

28. Echlin P (1974) Coating techniques for scanning electron microscopy. Scanning Electron Microsc 7:1019–1028

29. Holland VF (1976) Some artifacts associated with sputter-coated samples observed at high magnifications in the scanning electron microscope. Scanning Electron Microsc 9:71–74

30. Ingram P, Morosoff N, PopeL, Allen F, Tisher C (1976) Some comparisons of the techniques of sputter (coating) and evaporative coating for scanning electron microscopy. Scanning Electron Microsc 9:75–82

31. Boyde A, Wood C (1969) Preparation of animal tissues for surface-scanning electron microscopy. J Microsc 90:221–249

32. Murakami T (1974) A revised tannin-osmium method for non-coated scanning electron microscope specimens. Arch Histol Jap 36:189–193

33. Sasaki K (1988) A simple method to observe intracellular organelles with the scanning electron microscope. J Electron Microsc (Tokyo) 37:171–173

34. Boyde A (1972) Biological specimen preparation for the scanning electron microscope, a overview. Scanning Electron Microsc 5:257–264

35. Malick LE,Wilson RB (1975) Evaluation of a modified technique for SEM examination for vertebrate specimens without evaporated metal layers. Scanning Electron Microsc 8:259–266

36. Akahori I, Ishi H, Naka I, Yoshida H (1988) A simple freeze-drying device using t-butyl alcohol for SEM specimens. J Electron Microsc 37:351–352

37. Osatake H, Atom K, Mitsushima A, Tanak K (1980) A simple method of freeze-drying for scanning electron microscopy. J Electron Microsc (Tokyo) 29:72–74

38. Demsey A, Kawka D, Stackpole C (1978) Cell surface membrane organization revealed by freeze-drying. J Ultrastruct Res 62:13–25

39. Fujikawa S, Suzuki T, Ishikawa T, Sakurai S, Hasegawa Y (1988) Continuous observation of frozen biological material with cryo-scanning electron microscope and freeze-replica by a new cryo-system. J Electron Microsc (Tokyo) 37:315–322

40. Humphreys WJ, Spurlock BO, Johnson S (1974) Critical point drying of ethanol-infiltrated cryo-fractured biological specimens for scanning electron microscopy. Scanning Electron Microsc 7:275–282

41. Tokunaga J, Edanaga N, Fujita T, Adachi K (1974) Freeze cracking of scanning electron microscope specimens. A study of the kidney and spleen. Arch Histol Jap 37:165–182

42. Boyde A (1974) Freezing, freeze-fracturing and freeze-drying in biological specimen preparation for the SEM. Scanning Electron Microsc pp 1043–1046

43. Roth J, Meyer HW (1972) Electron microscopic studies in mammalian lungs by freeze-etching: III. The bronchiolar cells with special consideration of the Clara cells. Exp Pathol 7:71–83

44. Anderson PM (1979) The respiratory system. In: Hodges CM, Hallowes RC (eds) Biomedical research application of scanning electron microscopy, vol 1. London, pp 177–202

Chapter 2
Ciliated Cells of the Tracheobronchial Tree and Their Morphology on SEM

P. C. Braga and G. Piatti

Centro di Farmacologia Respiratoria, Facoltà di Medicina e Chirurgia,
Università degli Studi di Milano

With scanning electron microscopy one can examine the surface morphology and distribution of the epithelial cells of the airways.

The airways can be divided into different regions according to the distribution of the epithelial cell population: the trachea and extrapulmonary bronchi; the intrapulmonary bronchi (diameter > 500 μm); and the bronchioles (diameter < 500 μm). From their surface morphology, the cells lining the respiratory airways can be divided into ciliated cells and nonciliated cells. The latter include secretory cells (mucous, serous, and Clara cells), basal or intermediate cells, and brush cells, if present [1].

In the SEM, ciliated cells, where visible, are polygonal in outline, but this is appreciable only in particular situations, because they are densely covered with peculiar long processes called cilia. The extensive coverage of mucosa by cilia makes it difficult to see the intermingled nonciliated cells, whose apices randomly, and rarely, protrude beyond the ciliary fringe. The general aspect at low magnification resembles the Amazonian forest seen from an airplane, in which only the top of the trees are visible and, in our case, instead of leaves the cilia and their tips are visible.

Ciliated cells are roughly columnar and, together with goblet and basal cells, form a pseudostratified epithelium which covers the tracheo bronchial tree [2]. A typical epithelial cell bears about 200–250 cilia on its apical surface, but this number varies in different animals and at different levels of the respiratory tree. In the larger airways, the cilia extend 5–8 μm from the cell surface, but in some mammalian epithelia the cilia can be shorter. They are spaced uniformly along the cell surface and at their base, between adjacent cilia, it is possible to see the microvilli, which are small cylindrical extensions of the membrane, 0.1–0.2 μm long, that have been hypothesized as having a function in exchange mechanisms of the cell and in the reabsorption of excess fluid rising from the enormous surface of the distal airways to the smaller surface of the trachea [3, 4]. Table 1 lists some characteristics of cilia of the respiratory tract.

The tip of the cilium is not a smooth spherical surface, but has three to seven small clawlike projections protruding 250–600 Å from the surface. This microciliary crown has also been observed in oviduct [5] and in tracheal cilia of several animals, including frogs and humans [6–8]. In the mechanics of the cilium under normal conditions, only its tip enters the mucus layer for 5000–8000 Å. The microciliary crown may therefore be important for hooking the glycoprotein

Table 1. Characteristics of cilia of respiratory mucosa

Parameter	Dimensions
Length	5.0–8.0 μm
Diameter	0.15–0.3 μm
Cilia spacing	0.3–0.4 μm
Density of cilia	6.0–10/μm^2
Number of cilia per cell	200–400
Metachronism	antiplectic
Metachronal wavelength	20–40 μm
Frequency of beat	10–30 Hz
	(600–1800 beats/min)
Average velocity of mucus	5–10 mm/min
In trachea	5–20 mm/min
In terminal bronchioles	100–600 μm/min

fibrils in the ciliary beat which moves the mucus. Atypical cilia of various types can be found in apparently normal lungs and in disease states [9].

The axonema is the central portion of the cilium. It consists of nine microtubule doublets disposed in a circle around a central pair of single microtubules. Each of the nine outer microtubular doublets consists of an A and a B subfiber. Cilia beat about 600–1000 times per minute, the motility resulting from sliding of the axonemal microtubules [10–13]. The effective beat in the upper and lower respiratory tract is always toward the pharynx [9]. Mammalian cilia, like other cilia, have two kinds of movements, one an effective propulsive stroke and the other a recovery stroke. The recovery stroke continues into the effective stroke without pause and lasts nearly twice as long. Resting phases of different duration occur at the end of the effective stroke. The effective stroke is asymmetric and is predominantly vertical, while the recovery stroke is more horizontal [13]. This difference is the hydrodynamic basis for ciliary propulsion, because the effective stroke carries along with it a larger volume of material than the recovery stroke.

Respiratory tract cilia begin their beat cycle from a resting position, in which the cilia lie with their tips pointing toward the oropharynx, in the direction of flow of the mucus [14].

Cilia, both individually and together, produce a kinetic force, and theoretical approaches have been developed to calculate this force, so as to understand the limits beyond which the movement of mucus stops.

Raptis and Perdikis [15], and later Pui-Man Low [16], calculated the force *(F)* produced by a single cilium during its movement from the following equation:

$$F = 8\pi\mu(\bar{v} - \bar{u})a_0 \frac{L(1-\gamma)}{4} = h^2(\varrho g\delta) = 0.001 \text{ g s}^{-2}$$

where

$L(1-\gamma)$	= extrapolated length of a cilium
μ	= viscosity of medium
$\bar{u}$	= absolute mean velocity at the top of the cilia (313 ms^{-1})
δ	= thickness of the medium
h	= distance between cilia
a_0	= radius of the cilia
ϱ	= density of medium
γ	= 0.8
v	= 3.02×10^{-2} cm s^{-1}
g	= net force exerted by the cilium on the fluid

The result was $F \simeq 0.001$ g $\times$ s^{-2}, which corresponds to about 0.001 dyn. Barton and Raynor [17] used another equation

$$F_x = \frac{2S\omega(1-\gamma^2)L\mu}{\ln[\omega a S(1+\gamma)/4\pi v]} = 0.0006 \text{ cm g s}^{-2}$$

and calculated a force $F \simeq 0.0006$ dyn, about 40% less than that above.

Although this theoretical approach is interesting, it is not easy to transfer into clinical practice. The information can be understood better if we remember that experiments with frog palate have shown that ciliary transport still occurred when weights of up to 20 mg/mm^2 were put on the ciliated epithelium [18].

With cryofracture we can obtain a view of the lateral surface of ciliated cells, showing their relationships to other cells of the pseudostratified tissue. This topic is of interest to a large audience of investigators, and data have been published on morphological features of airway surface epithelial cells in different animals, including amphibians [19], frog [20], chicken [21], rat [22, 23], guinea pig [24], rabbit [25, 26], dog [27], monkey [28], other mammalian species [29, 30], and man [31–38].

Acknowledgements. The authors thank Raven Press, New York, for permission to reproduce the micrographs in Figs. 2.13 and 2.14 and Table 1 from Guffanti EE, Vercelloni SM, Piatti G, Braga PC (1990) Cilia and mucociliary Clearance. In: Allegra L, Braga PC (eds) Bronchial Mucology and related diseases. Raven, New York, 1990, pp 29–30.

References

1. Souma T (1987) The distribution and surface ultrastructure of airways epithelial cells in the rat lung: a scanning electron microscopic study. Arch Histol Jap 50:419–436
2. Tandler B, Sherman JM, Boat T (1983) Surface architecture of the mucosae epithelium of the cat. Trachea I, cartilaginous portion. Am J Anat 168:119–131
3. Bennet HS (1963) Morphological aspects of extracellular polysaccharides. J Histochem Cytochem 11:14–23
4. Kilburn KH (1968) A hypothesis for pulmonary clearance and its implications. Am Rev Respir Dis 48:449–463

5. Foroglou-Kerameos C, Mantos A, Bontis I, Katsaros I (1983) Présence de microcils sur l'extremité apicale des cils de l'épithelium de la trompe uterine. Acta Anat (Basel) 115:107–116

6. Kuhn C, Engleman W (1978) The structure of the tips of mammalian respiratory cilia. Cell Tissue Res 186:491–498

7. Foliguet B, Puchelle E (1986) Apical structure of human respiratory cilia. Bull Eur Physiopathol Respir 22:43–47

8. Le Cluyse EL, Dentler WL (1984) Asymmetrical microtubule capping structures in frog palate cilia. J Ultrastruct Res 86:75–85

9. Breeze R, Tork M (1984) Cellular structure, function and organization in the lower respiratory tract. Environ Health Perspect 35:3–24

10. Afzeliûs BA (1983) Ultrastructural basis for ciliary motility. Eur J Respir Dis 64 (Suppl 128):280–286

11. Horridge GA, Tamm SL (1969) Critical Point drying for scanning electron microscopic study of ciliary motion. Science 163:817–818

12. Satir PI (1968) Studies on cilia: III. Further studies on the cilium tip and a "sliding filament" model of ciliary motility. J Cell Biol 39:77–94

13. Rautiainen MEP (1988) Orientation of human respiratory cilia. Eur Respir J 1:257–261

14. Sanderson HJ, Dirksen ER, Satir P (1990) Electron microscopy of respiratory tract cilia. In: Schraufragel DE (ed) Electron microscopy of the lung. Dekker, New York, pp 47–69

15. Raptis A, Perdikis C (1983) A mathematical model of the cilia for pharyngeal epithelium of the frog. J Biomech 16:235–236

16. Pui-Man Low P (1984) A modified mathematical model of the cilia for pharingeal epithelium of the frog. J Biomech 17:815

17. Barton C, Raynor S (1967) Analytical investigation of cilia induced mucous flow. Bull Math Biophys 29:419–428

18. Stewart WC (1948) Weight-carrying capacity and excitability of excised ciliated epithelium. Am J Physiol 152:1–5

19. Hard R, Rieder CL (1983) Mucociliary transport in new lungs: the ultrastructure of the ciliary apparatus in isolated epithelial sheets and in functional triton-extracted models. Tissue Cell 15:227–243

20. Puchelle E, Petit A, Adnet JJ (1984) Fine structure of the frog palate mucociliary epithelium. J Submicrosc Cytol 16:273–282

21. Reissig M, Bang BG, Bang BF (1978) Ultrastructure of the mucociliary interface in the nasal mucosa of the chicken. Am Rev Respir Dis 117:327–341

22. Smolich JJ, Stratford BF, Maloney JE, Ritchie B (1976) Postnatal development of the epithelium of larinx and trachea in the rat: scanning electron microscopy. J Anat 124:657–673

23. McAteer J (1984) Tracheal morphogenesis and fetal development of the mucociliary epithelium of the rat. Scanning Electron Microsc 4:1995–2008

24. Dalen H (1983) An ultrastructural study of the tracheal epithelium of the guinea-pig with special reference to the ciliary structure. J Anat 136:46–67

25. Kennedy JR, Ranyard JR (1983) Morphology and quantitation of ciliated outgrowths from cultured rabbit tracheal explants. Eur J Cell Biol 29:200–208

26. Barber VC, Boyde A (1968) Scanning electron microscopic studies of cilia. Z Zellforsch 84:269–284

27. Wright NG, Brown RMH, McCandlish IAP, Thompson H, Cornwell HJC (1983) Patterns of cilia formation in the lower respiratory tract of dog: a scanning electron microscopic study. Res Vet Sci 34:340–346

28. Castleman WL, Dungworth DL, Tyler WS (1975) Intrapulmonary airway morphology in three species of monkeys. A correlated scanning and transmission electron microscopic study. Am J Anat 142:107–122

29. Plopper CG, Mariassy AT, Wilson DW, Alley JL, Nisho SJ, Nettersheim P (1983) Comparison of nonciliated tracheal epithelial cells in six mammalian species: ultrastructure and population densities. Exp Lung Res 5:281–294

30. Greenwood MF, Holland P (1972) The mammalian respiratory tract surface. A scanning electron microscopic study. Lab Invest 27:296–304

31. Jeffery PK (1983) Morphologic features of airway surface epithelial cells and glands. Am Rev Respir Dis 128:14–20

32. Kessel RG, Kardon RH (1979) Tissues and organs, a text-atlas of scanning electron microscopy. Freeman New York

33. Moscoso GJ, Nandra K, Driver M (1989) Ciliogenesis and ciliation of the respiratory epithelium in the human fetal cartilaginous trachea. Path Res Pract 184:161–167

34. Moscoso GJ, Driver M, Codd J, Whimstr WF (1988) The morphology of ciliogenesis in the developing fetal human respiratory epithelium. Pathol Res Pract 183:403–411

35. Jeffery PK, Brain APR (1988) Surface morphology of human airway mucosa, normal, carcinoma or cystic fibrosis. Scanning Microsc 2:553–560

36. Boysen M (1982) The surface structure of the human nasal mucosa. Virchows Arch [B] 40:279–294

37. Roessler F, Grossenbacher R, Walt H (1988) Effects of tracheostomy on human tracheobronchial mucosa: a scanning electron microscopic study. Laryngoscope 98:1261–1267

38. Andrews PM (1979) The respiratory system. In: Hodges GM, Hallowes RC (eds) Biomedical research applications of SEM, vol I. Academic, New York, pp 177–202

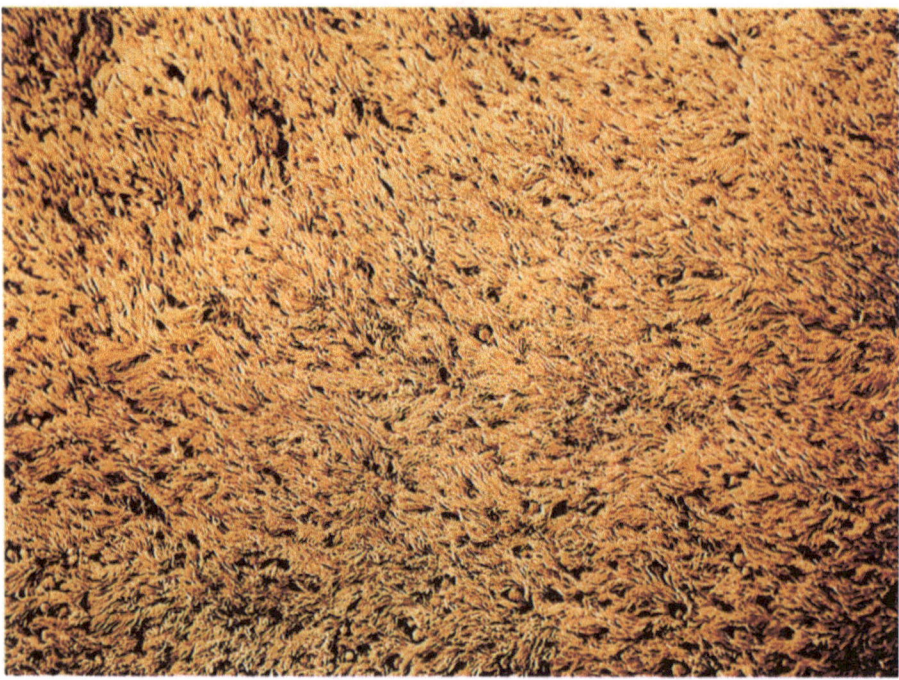

Fig. 2.1. Scanning electron micrograph at low power (×356) showing the surface of a normal tracheal epithelium. The cilia of ciliated cells form a homogeneous carpetlike surface punctuated by small areas of discontinuity hiding occasional nonciliated cells

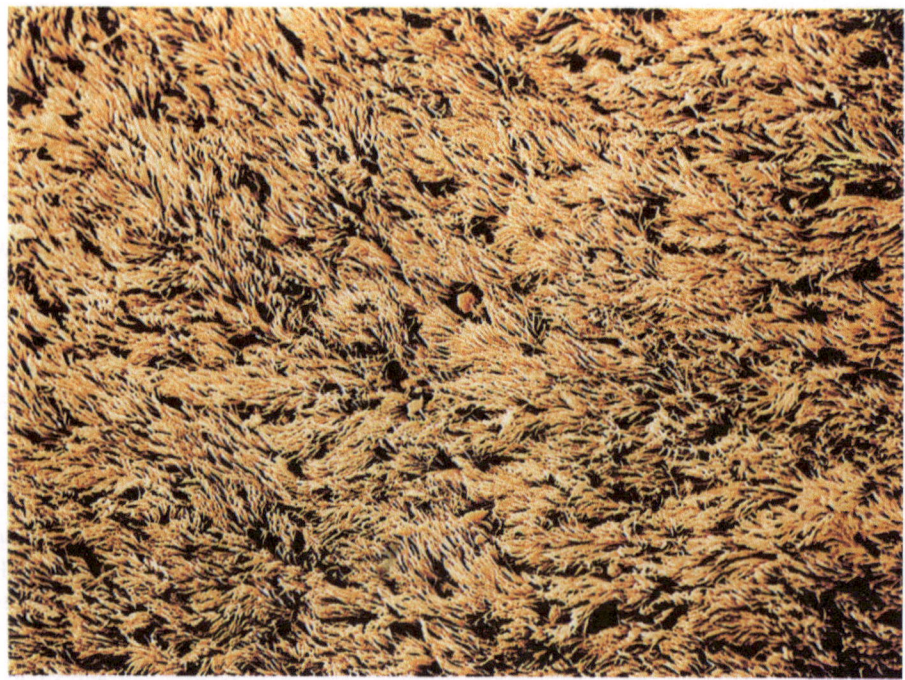

Fig. 2.2. Enlarging the above picture (×660), bundles of individual cilia orientied in this case from right to left, became visible

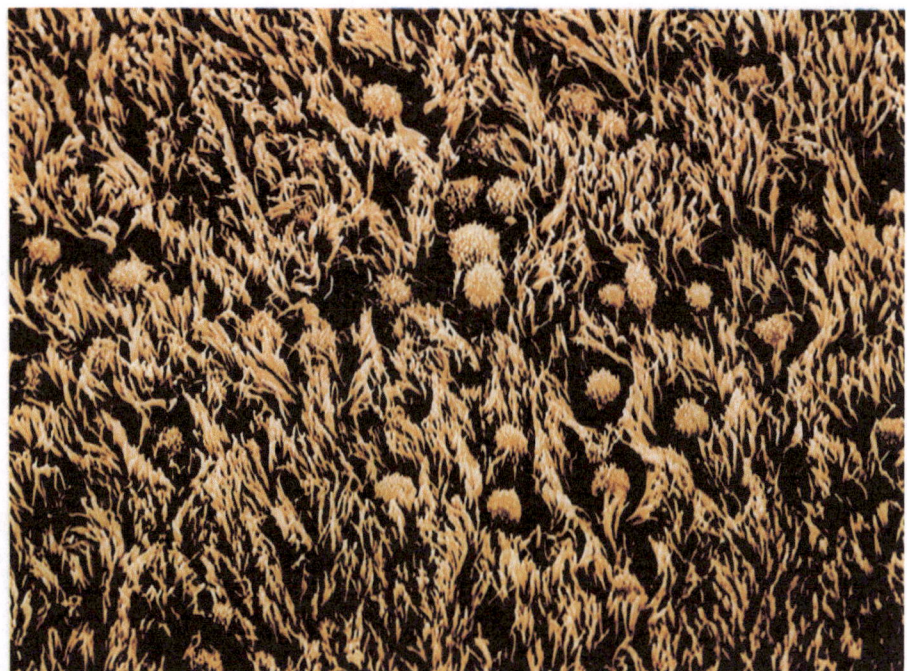

Fig. 2.3. Scanning electron micrograph showing the carpet formed by ciliated cells in a 2nd-order human bronchus. At this magnification (×1050), the nonciliated cells are now visible in the form of small spherical formations randomly distributed. The ratio between ciliated and nonciliated cells is generally 5:1, but it can vary greatly from one part of the tracheobronchial tree to another even in healthy lungs and more so in pathological conditions

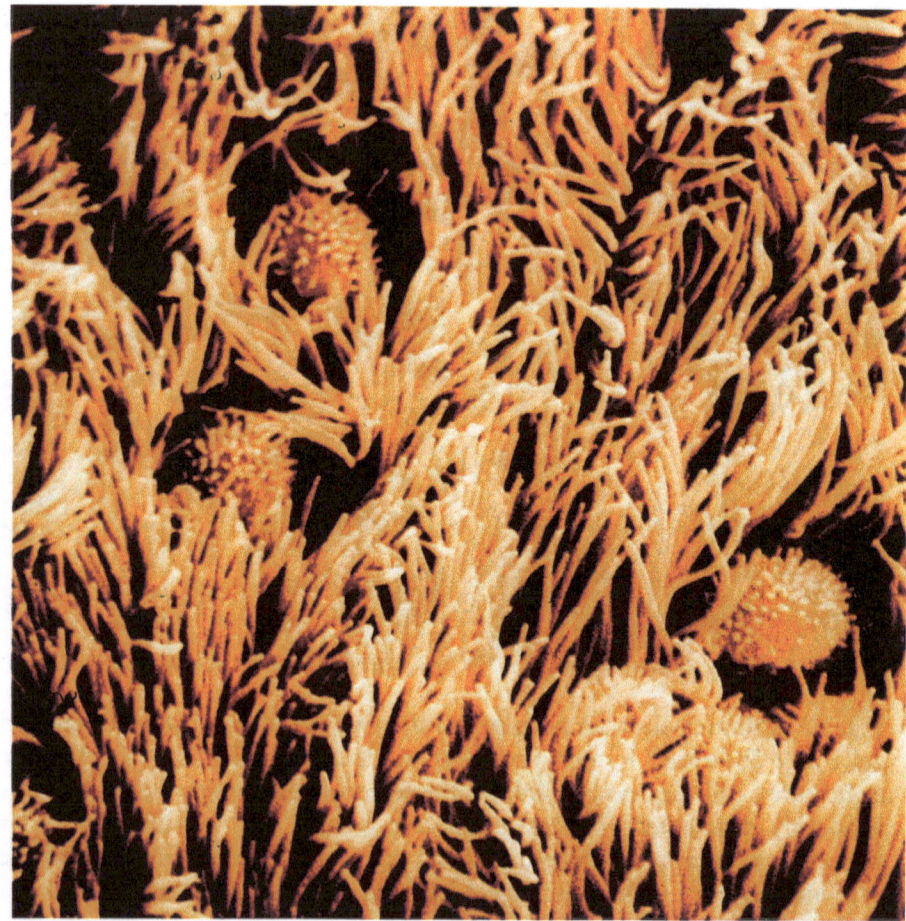

Fig. 2.4. This picture shows the appearance of the surface of a region of trachea at a magnification of ×2600. At the *top left* and *bottom right* some goblet cells are present

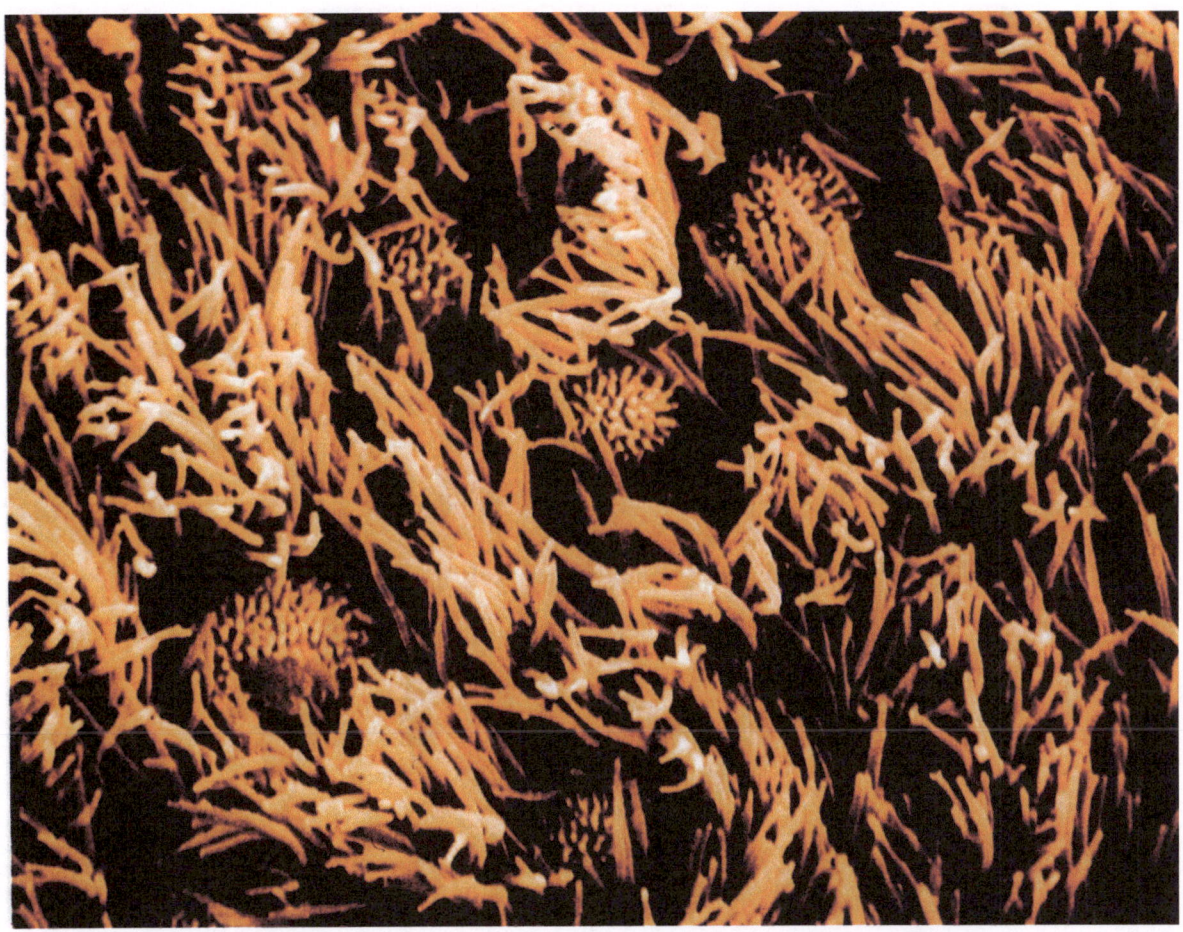

Fig. 2.5. The surface of a bronchus (×3860). The close similarity between this and Fig. 2.4. is obvious, both showing the type of epithelium lining the respiratory mucosa of extrapulmonary bronchi. With some modification, this epithelium covers the mucosa up to the last intrapulmonary bronchi

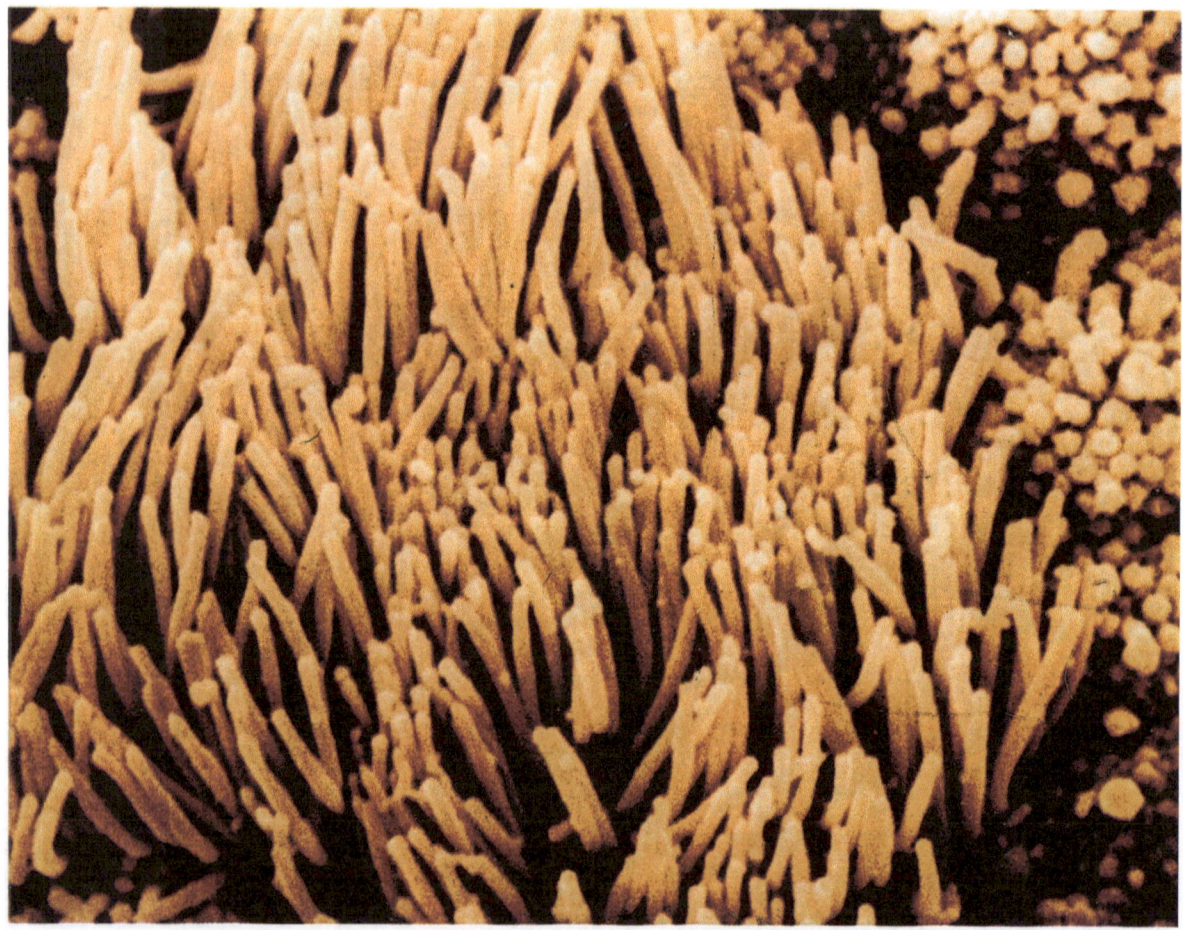

Fig. 2.6. Each ciliated cell is covered by an average of 100–200 cilia. In this picture the density of the closely packed cilia is well depicted (×4400)

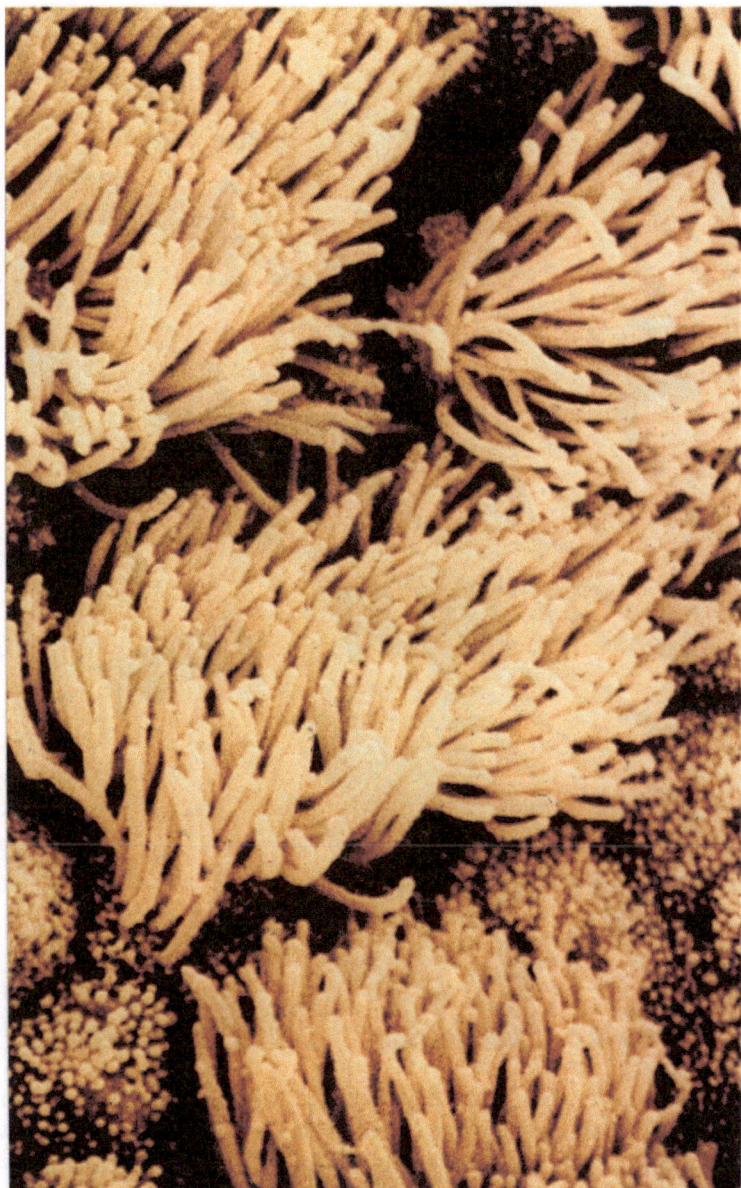

Fig. 2.7. Another view of the morphology of the ciliated cells
(×4200)

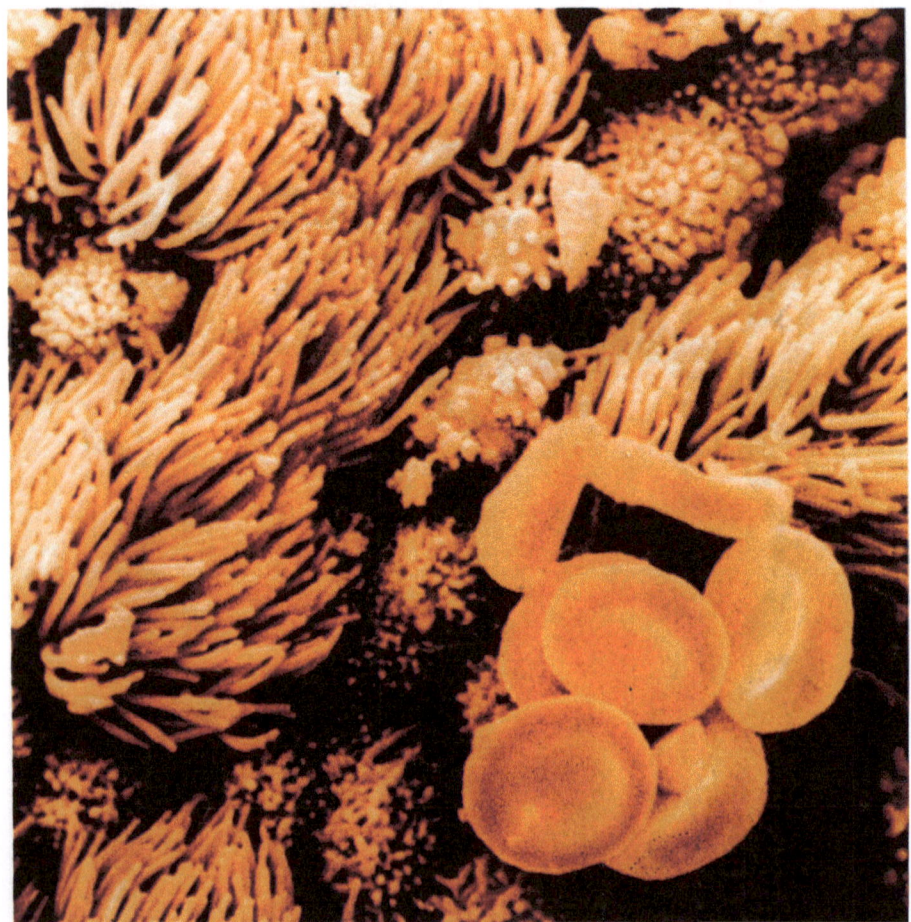

Fig. 2.8. In the *lower right* some erythrocytes, while in the *upper left* there are ciliated cells. The diameter of the erythrocytes is on average 5–7 μm, which is about the same as the length of the cilia, which are long on average 4–7 μm (×2500)

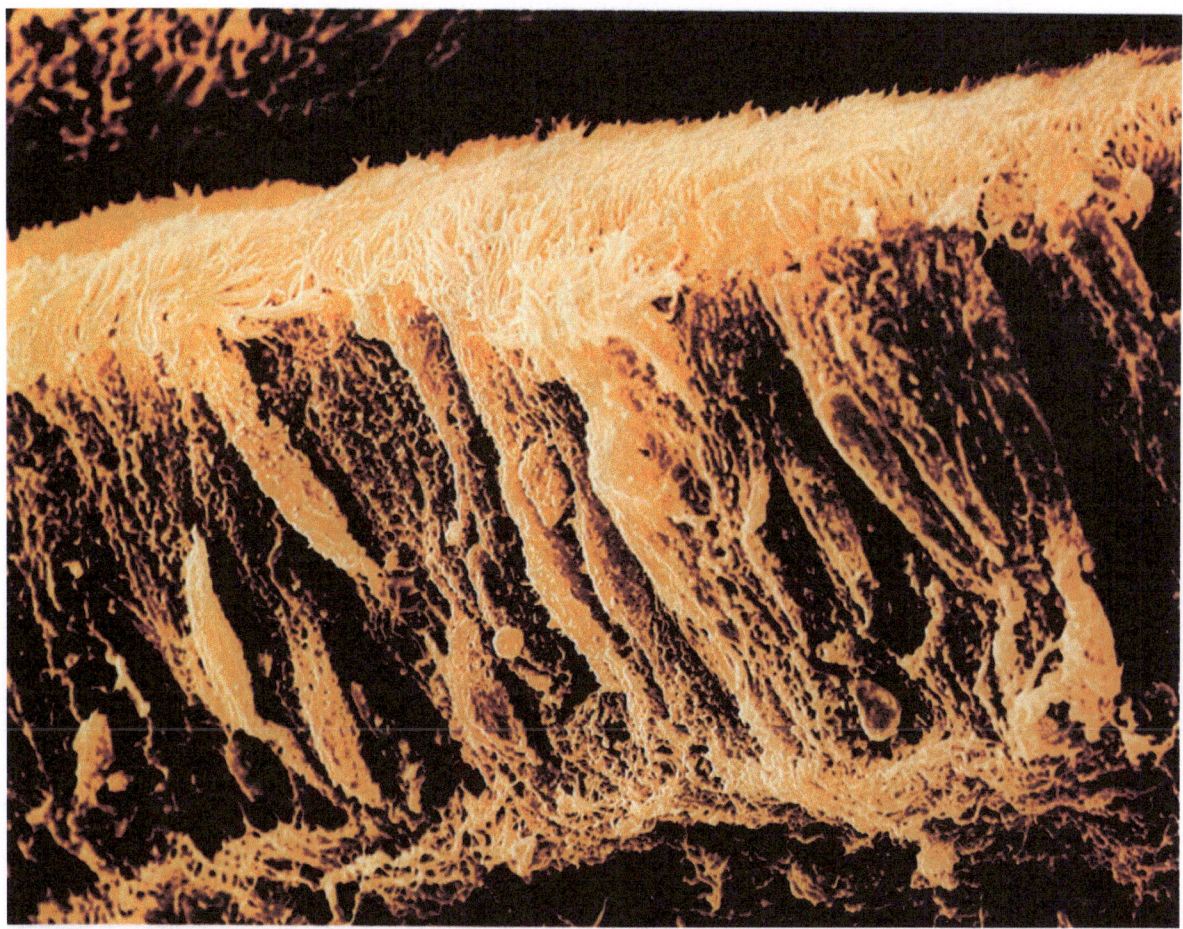

Fig. 2.9. Epithelial edge of human trachea obtained by freeze-fracture showing both a lateral and a surface view of the normal pseudostratified structure. The columnar structure formed by narrow bodies of the ciliated cells is clear. These cells reside on a basement membrane which appears as network of small connective filaments (reticular laminae) belonging to the lamina propria. Small basal cells are also present within the columnar epithelium at various locations (×1150)

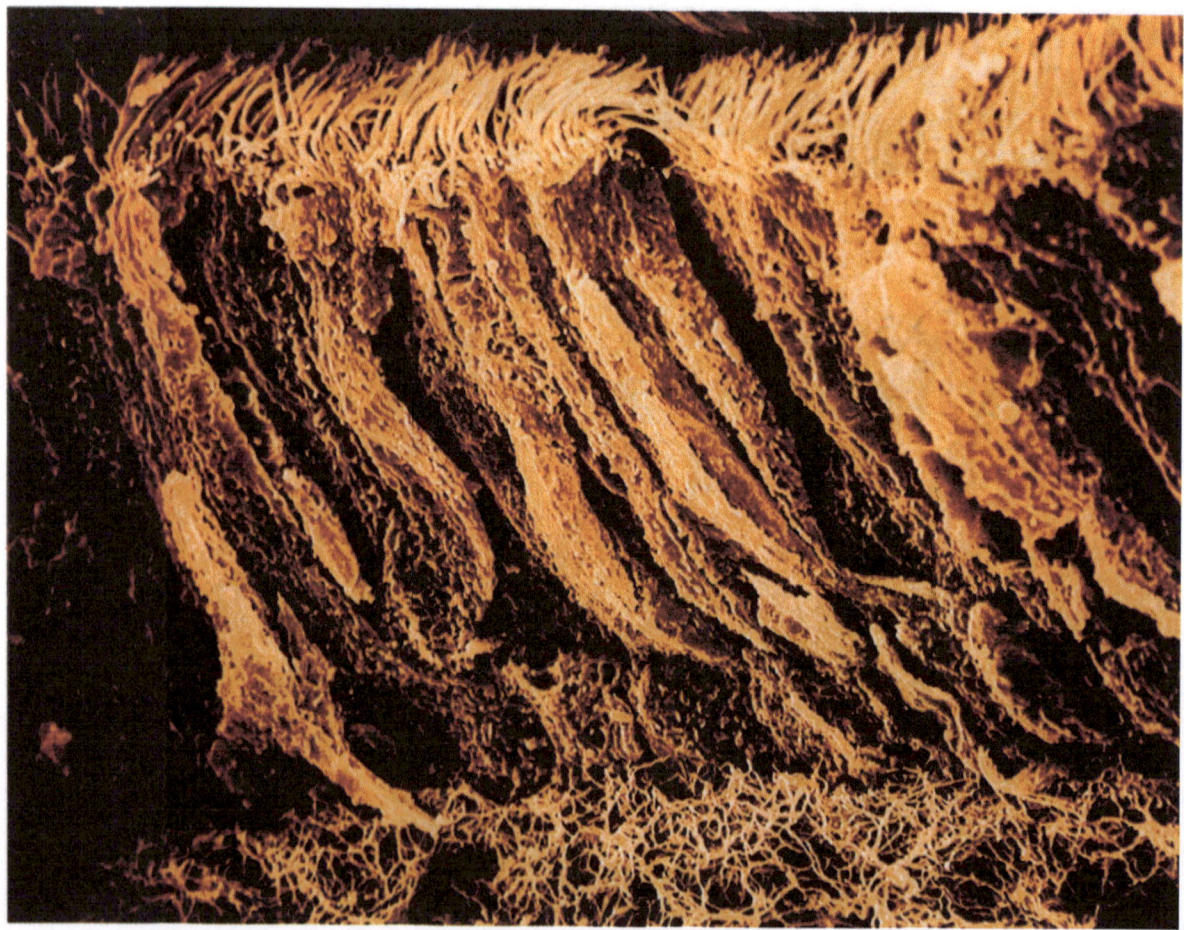

Fig. 2.10. The appearance of this micrograph is similar to that of the above scanning electron micrograph in Fig. 2.9 although the tissue sample was from a bronchus (×1555). These two figures have been selected to shown only ciliated cells. In other fractures goblet cells are also present

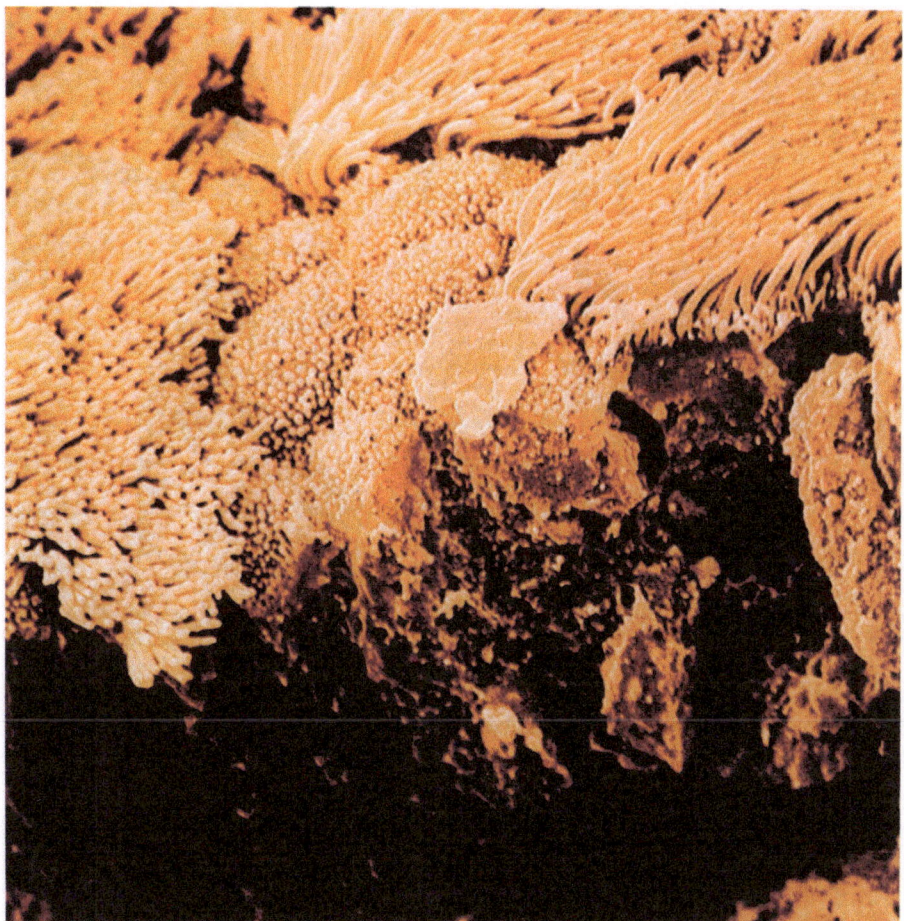

Fig. 2.11. Surface epithelium seen "on edge" at a different angle from Figs. 2.9 and 2.10, showing simultaneously the top and the side surfaces of ciliated cells. Some goblet cells are also present (×1850)

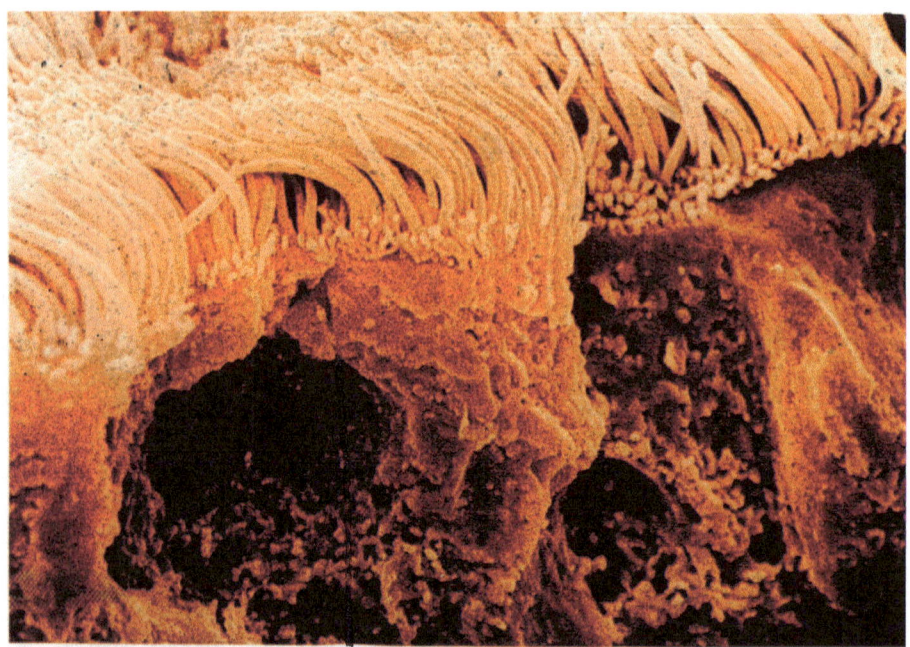

Fig. 2.12. In this freeze-cracking preparation, seen at higher magnification than the others (×4000), it is possible to observe a negative cast of a goblet cell, easily identifiable by the round body shape, which is clearly different from the narrow long shape of the body of ciliated cells (see Figs. 2.9, 2.10). Note the presence of many surface processes smaller than cilia located at the base of ciliated cells. These processes are called microvilli

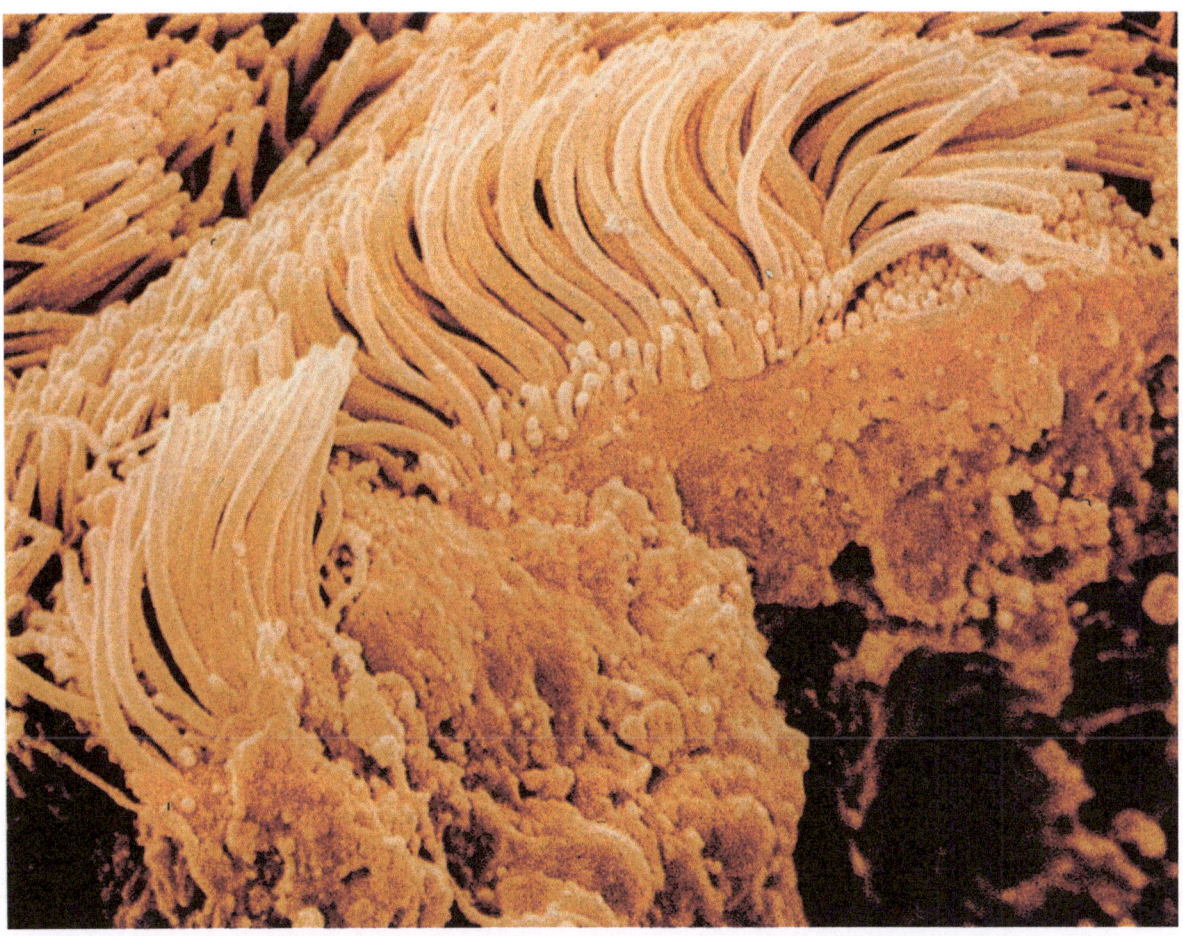

Fig. 2.13. Another view of the lateral aspect of cracked epithelium. In this case, along with microvilli, it is also possible to see a row of cilia, with progressively different degrees of bending, as they were frozen during their movements. Bending happens during the recovery cycle ($\times$5000)

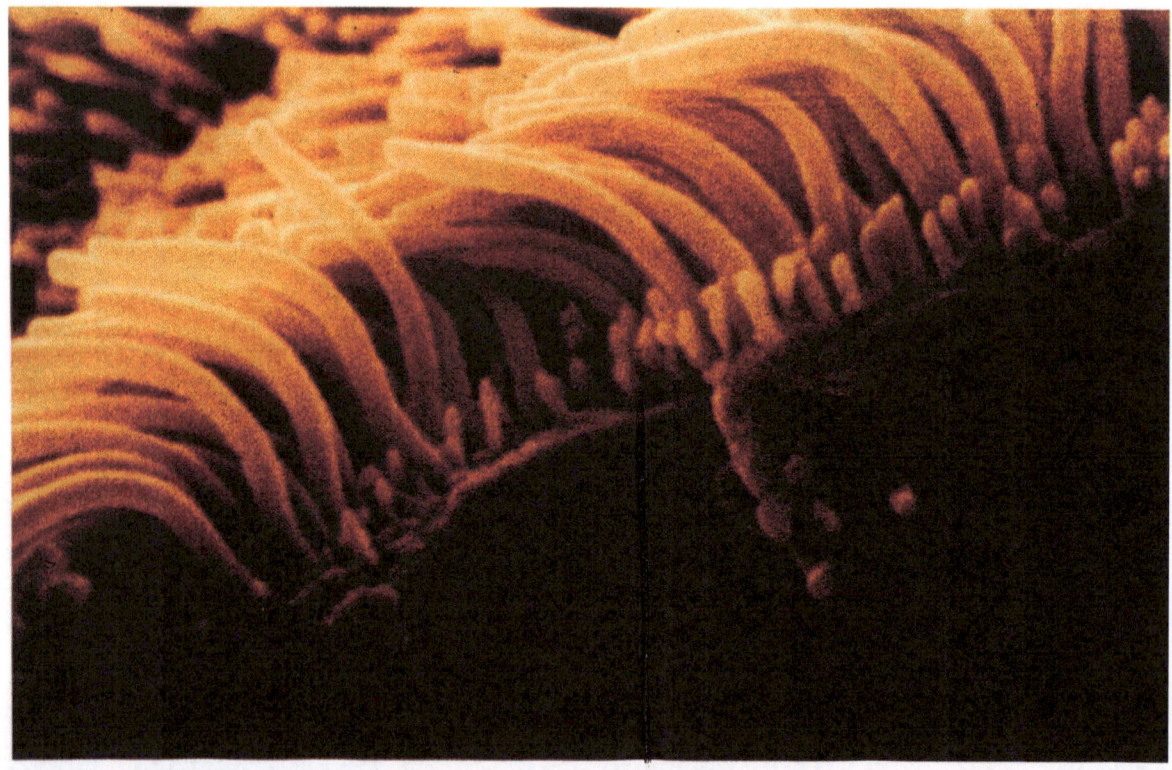

Fig. 2.14. This micrograph is at ×9150 to show the relative dimensions and
relationships between cilia and microvilli

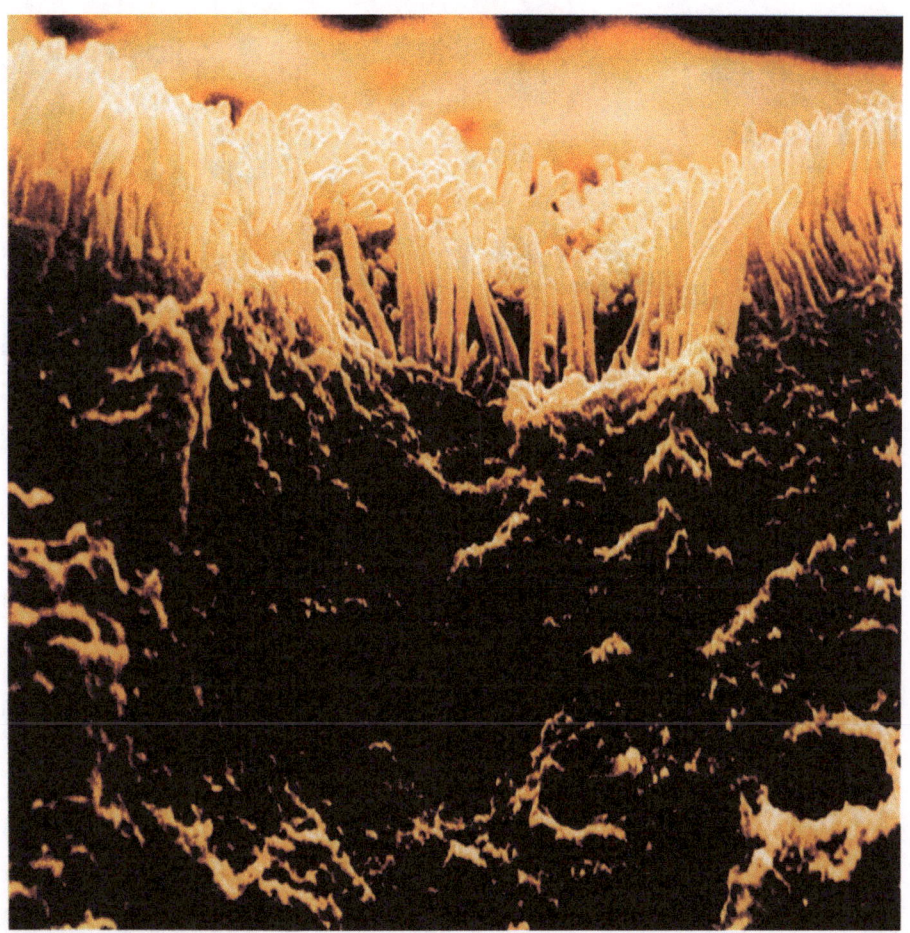

Fig. 2.15. This is an "unusual" view of a fractured epithelium. Generally, the specimens are viewed from the top surface or laterally; in this case the view is from bottom to top (×2100)

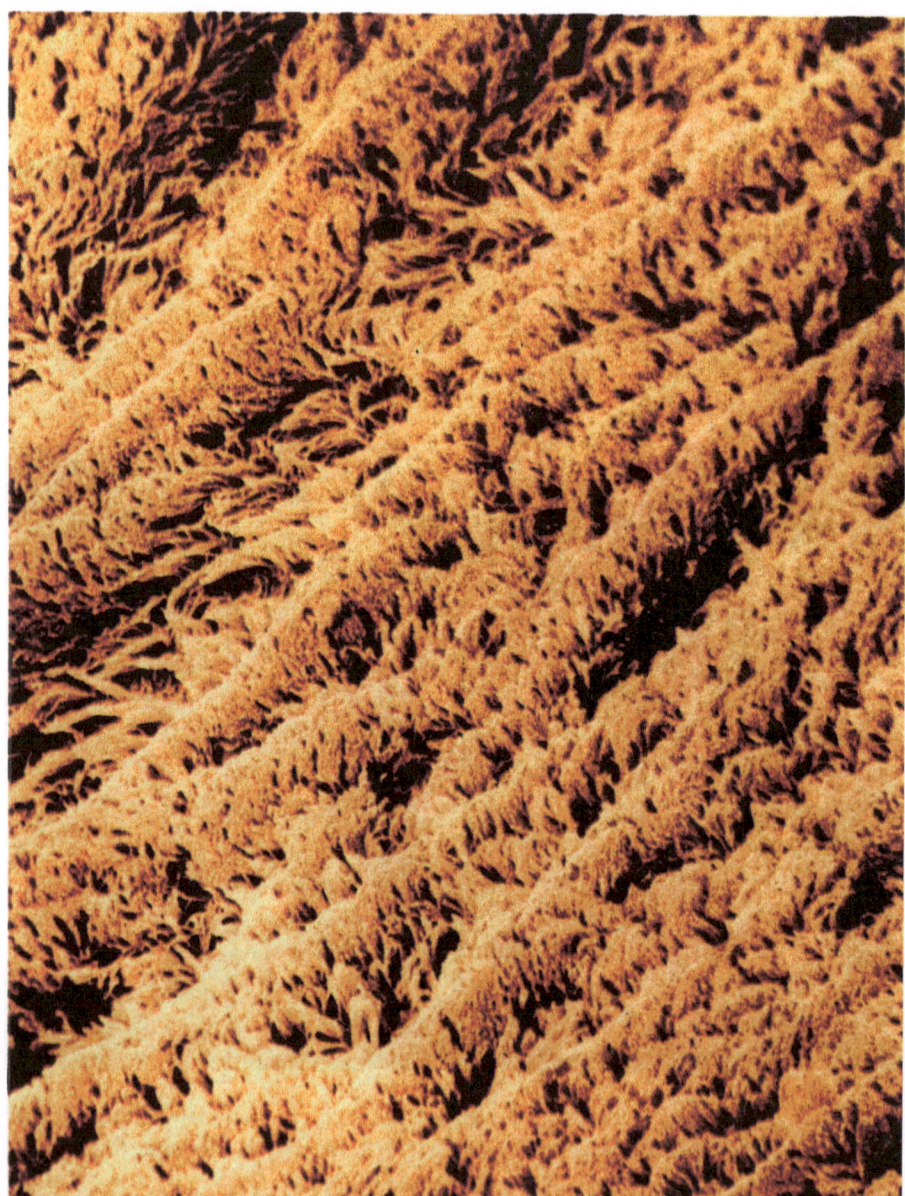

Fig. 2.16. This specimen is from a frog palate and has been selected to show the synchronized methacronal waves of the ciliated epithelium (×680)

Chapter 3
Morphological Aspects of Mucus Lining the Airways and of the Cells That Secrete It

P. C. Braga and G. Piatti

Centro di Farmacologia Respiratoria, Facoltà di Medicina e Chirurgia,
Università degli Studi di Milano

"Mucus" is the name of an extracellular material that lines the epithelium of the trachea, extrapulmonary bronchi, and intrapulmonary bronchi generally up to a diameter of 500 μm. Mucus is basically a mixture of apocrine secretions from secretory cells of respiratory mucosa and submucosal glands [1-3], but it also contains cells (nonresident) and other material present in the breathed air. The expectorated mucus (sputum) is mixed with saliva, cells, and material from the nose, pharynx, and mouth.

Mucus serves as an interface between inspired/expired air and the respiratory mucosa and, since it lines the airways, provides the first and main line of defense against inhaled pollutants. Mucus has specific physicochemical characteristics that enable it to trap noxious exogenous inorganic and organic matter (in gaseous, liquid, or solid form), which can then be removed by the mucociliary clearance mechanism. This mechanism provides for the flow of mucus lining the airways towards the head by the propulsive force of the underlying ciliated cells [4, 5].

There is continous secretion of mucus onto the luminal surface of the airway mucosa. This extracellular material comes from the two sources: individual epithelial serous and goblet cells, which are scattered throughout the pseudostratified epithelium covering the airways; and the mucous glands, which are tubular acinar glands located in the airway wall, with ducts opening into the bronchial lumen [1]. In healthy humans, there is an average of one gland per square millimeter of trachea [6].

It is not known why there are two different sources for mucus secretion. One hypothesis is that in normal conditions goblet cells more rapidly release mucus, perhaps with high molecular weight mucins, while the gland cells release mucus more slowly, perhaps with lower molecular weight mucins. In any case, since the total volume of mucous glands has been estimated to be about 40 times that of goblet cells, it is assumed the goblet cells produce 1/40 of the final amount of mucus. Findings from functional and structural studies of airway epithelia indicate the mucus and serous cells to be the predominant nonciliated secretory cells of proximal conducting airways (trachea and bronchi) and the Clara cells to be the secretory cells of the distal conducting airways (bronchioles) [7-9].

Chemically, mucus is 95% water, 3% protein, 1% lipid, and 1% inorganic matter. The protein and glycoprotein content, which varies according to physiological or pathological conditions, governs the physical and rheological properties of the secretion. The glycoproteins are proteins with polylypeptide backbones covalently linked to repeating oligosaccharide side chains containing sialic acid and sulfate, which can be identified by histochemical techniques [10].

The surfaces of goblet cells are characterized by the presence of short microvilli, approximately 0.2-1.0 μm long and about 0.1 μm diameter. These microvilli can vary in dimension and number, depending the secretory phase of the goblet. Cells in the early stages of secretion are almost completely covered by microvilli.

The process of accumulation of mucus in the apical part of the goblet cells is accompanied by a decrease in the number and dimensions of microvilli. Later, the microvilli disappear completely and the apical surface of the goblet cells, which may protrude into the tracheal lumen above the level of the adjacent cilia, becomes dome-shaped; sometimes the shapes of the secretory granules are visible under the membrane [4, 11]. Mucus is secreted by goblet cells through rupture of the cell surface and by release of granules at the cell apex, which after discharge may become flattened or collapsed into a crypt like structure [4, 11].

In chronic hypersecretory states, the tracheobronchial epithelium shows hyperplasia and hypertrophy of goblet cells and enlargement of submucosal glands in scattered areas of varying size. In specimens in which the lateral plasmalemma has been fortuitously cracked off, the outline of the goblet cells shows a broad apex and a narrow stemlike base, and the internal mucous droplets are clearly revealed.

In 1934, Lucas and Douglas [12] proposed that the fluid lining the respiratory mucosa is not homogenous, but that the layer closer to the epithelial cell surface (ciliated and nonciliated periciliary zone) is more fluid (sol-hypophase) and that the fluid gradually becomes thicker and more viscous and rich in mucous glycoprotein (gel-epiphase) closer to the luminal surface [13]. This double-layer model, in which cilia are beating in the watery hypophase and their tips are moving the gel layer of the epiphase, is still accepted today. What is visualized by SEM is the gel layer, also called the mucous blanket, because the sol layer is generally not retained and collapses during fixation and the dehydration maneuvers used to prepare the specimen for SEM observation.

Some investigators [14–16] who have studied mucus have suggested that the mucous layer covering the tracheobronchial tree is not a continous layer, but is in the form of streams, droplets, flakes, plaques of varying sizes. On the other hand, other investigators [17–19] have interpreted their findings in terms of a continuous mucous blanket with only some small holes or partial interruptions or discontinuities [20]. Certainly the technical procedure of specimen preparation for SEM observation (involving mechanical stress, fixation, dehydration, critical point drying) makes it very difficult to preserve the structure of the mucus present in wet physiological conditions [21, 22]. What we

see with SEM depends strictly on the amount of artifacts introduced, because the physicochemical characteristics and highly hydrated nature of mucus ensure that some unknown amount of shrinkage and artifacts will always be present [23–25]. In studying mucus and its relationships with the underlying tissues, in situ double fixation of the tissue by vascular perfusion [21, 26] and vapor fixation are to be preferred to the usual fixation by immersion. Obviously, no preventive lavage of the specimen should be performed.

In secretory cells, the products of secretion are stored in the form of small droplets, as can be seen by SEM and TEM, and during or immediately after the release of the secretion products, structures like droplets, small flakes, or plaques can be seen. In a later phase of ciliary mobilization and cephalad distribution these small amounts join in a more or less continuous mucus blanket.

It has also been observed that the thickness of the mucous layer is variable, being greater in the trachea (5–15 μm) and less in small lobar bronchi 1–4 μm). In the latter, the mucous blanket becomes thinner and is characterized by more open networks of fine fibrils and narrow interfibrillar spaces [19]. It must be remembered that the thickness of mucus at a site depends primarily [5, 19] on the amount of mucus produced and on its characteristics and its state of mobilization. Since observations with SEM are of necessity made on a limited area of a few square micrometers, it seems reasonable from a theoretical point of view to suppose that during the mobilization from small bronchi to larger ones, there is some spreading of mucus. Large areas of continous mucous blanket will form, but at the same time there will also be areas of thinning, or holes or discontinuities, of the blanket due to the natural inhomogeneity of the spreading mechanism. This inhomogeneity may result from many factors, such as different ciliated cell distribution, different cilia movement, or differences in the amount of mucus secretion. When interpreting findings from optical or electron microscopy (SEM or TEM) about the condition of mucus one should always remember these variability factors and not make absolute statements that could not correspond to reality.

References

1. Breeze R, Turk M (1984) Cellular structure, function and organization in the lower respiratory tract. Environ Health Perspect 55:3–24
2. Iravani J, Melville GN, Richter HG (1976) Mucus production influences by drugs: an electron microscopic study. Pneumologie 153 (Suppl):267–273
3. Ebert RV, Terracio MJ (1975) Observation of the secretion on the surface of the bronchioles with the scanning electron microscope. Am Rev Respir Dis 112:391–496
4. Sturgess JM, Czegledy-Nagy E (1978) Mucus secretion in the lung. Scanning Electron Microsc 2:1083–1088
5. Luchtel DL (1978) The mucous layer of the trachea and major bronchi in the rat. Scanning Electron Microsc 2:1089–1095
6. Widdicombe JG (1978) Control of secretion of tracheobronchial mucus. Br Med Bull 34:57–61
7. Reid L, Jones R (1979) Bronchial mucosal cells. Fed Proc 38:191–196
8. Breeze RG, Wheeldon EB (1977) The cells of the pulmonary airways. Am Rev Respir Dis 116:705–777
9. Plopper CG, Mariassy AT, Wilson DW, Alley JL, Nishio SJ, Nettesheim P (1983) Comparison of nonciliated tracheal epithelial cells in six mammalian species: ultrastructure and population densities. Exp Lung Res 5:281–294
10. Roussel P, Lamblin G, Houdfret N, Lhermitte M, Slayter HS (1984) Conformation of human mucus glycoproteins observed by electron microscopy. Biochem Soc Trans 12:617–618
11. Boysen M (1982) The surface structure of the human nasal mucosa: I. Ciliated and metaplasic epithelium in normal individual. A correlated study by scanning/transmission electron and light microscopy. Virchows Arch [B] 40:279–294
12. Lucas AM, Douglas LG (1934) Principles underlying ciliary activity in the respiratory tract: II. A comparison of nasal clearance in man, monkey and other mammals. Arch Otolaryngol 20:518–541
13. Asmundsson T, Kilburn KH (1973) Mechanism of respiratory tract clearance. In: Dulfano MJ (ed) Sputum: Fundamentals and clinical pathology. Thomas, Springfield, pp 107–180
14. Iravani J, Van As A (1972) Mucus transport in the tracheo-bronchial tree of normal and bronchitic rats. J Pathol 106:81–93
15. Van As A, Webster I (1974) The morphology of mucus in mammalian pulmonary airways. Environ Res 7:11–12
16. Van As A (1977) Pulmonary airway clearance mechanism: a reappraisal (editorial) Am Rev Respir Dis 115:721–726
17. Sturgess JM (1977) Structural organization of mucus in the lung. In: Sauders CL, Schneider RP, Dagle GE, Ragan HA (eds) Pulmonary macrophages and epithelial cells. National Technical Information Service, Springfield, pp 149–161
18. Sturgess JM (1977) The mucous lining of major bronchi in the rabbit lung. Am Rev Respir Dis 115:819–827
19. Sturgess JM (1978) Electron microscopy investigation of mucus. In: Braga PC, Allegra (eds) Methods in bronchial mucology. New York, pp 245–253
20. Yoneda K (1976) Mucus blanket of rat bronchus. An ultrastructural study. Am Rev Respir Dis 114:837–842
21. Garland CD, Nash GV, McMeekin JA (1982) The preservation of mucus and surface-associated microorganisms using acrolein vapor fixation. J Microscopy 128:307–312
22. Hulbert WC, Forster BB, Laird W, Phil CE, Walker DC (1982) An improved method for fixation of the respiratory epithelial surface with the mucous and surfactant layers. Lab Invest 47:354–363
23. Jenssen AO, Harbitz O, Smidsrod O (1980) Electron microscopy of mucin from sputum in chronic obstructive bronchitis. Eur J Respir Dis 61:71–76
24. Kory RC, Pendharker MB, Siegesmund KA, Pederson HJ, Boren HG (1970) Electron microscopy of sputum. Am Rev Respir Dis 101:385–394
25. Flood PR (1981) On the ultrastructure of mucus. Biomed Res 2:49–53
26. Gil J, Weibel ER (1969) Improvements in demonstration of lining layer of lung alveoli by electron microscopy. Respir Physiol 8:13–36

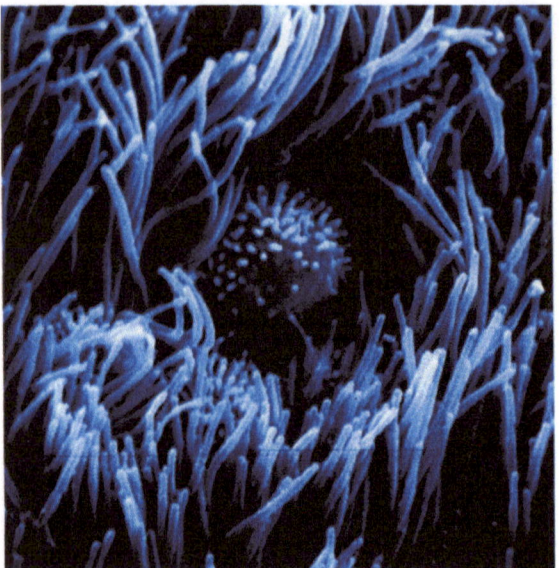

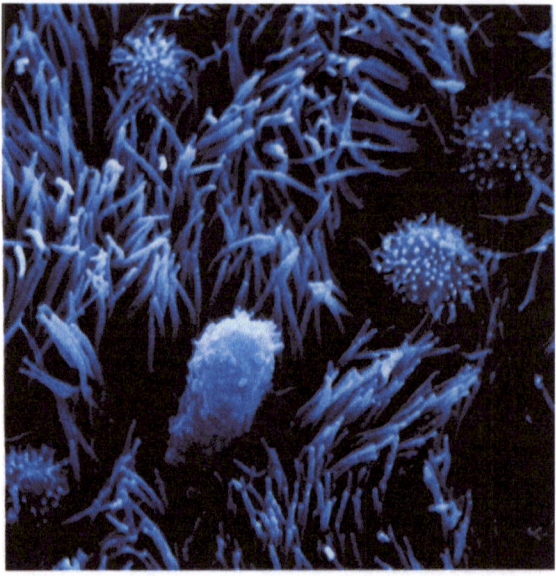

Fig. 3.1.a Tracheal epithelium. A scanning electron micrograph showing the appearance of a goblet cell rounded by cilia. The apical surface is dome-shaped and has small short processes called microvilli (×5200)

Fig. 3.1.b In the tracheal epithelium the goblet cells are randomly distributed among ciliated cells. In the *center* a goblet cell is protruding above the level of adjacent cilia, indicating an advanced phase of the mucus secretion process, while other goblet cells are not secreting and their surfaces are characterized by short microvilli (×4020)

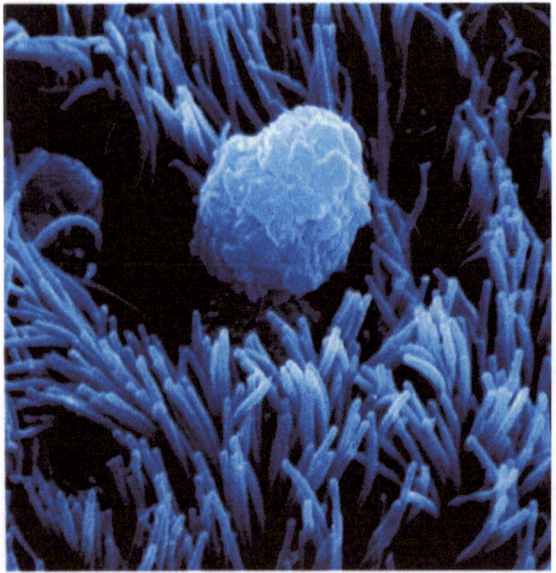

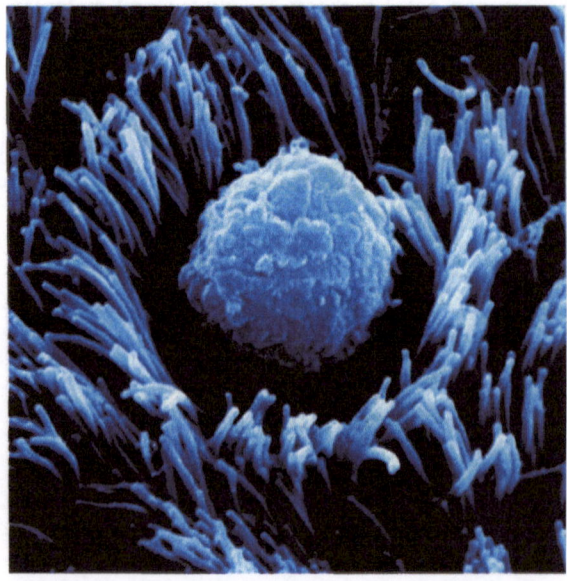

Fig. 3.1.c Main bronchus. The micrograph shows goblet cell during an advanced phase of the mucus secreting process. The microvilli are not present because the membrane which still covers the mucus is now very thin. It is possible to see details of the internal granular structure. Even the dome-shape of the apical part is lost and the upper part of the goblet cell protrudes over the cilia (×5200)

Fig. 3.1.d Main bronchus. This micrograph shows a further step in the growth of the apical portion of a goblet cell that is pushing the cilia to form a crown around it (×5700)

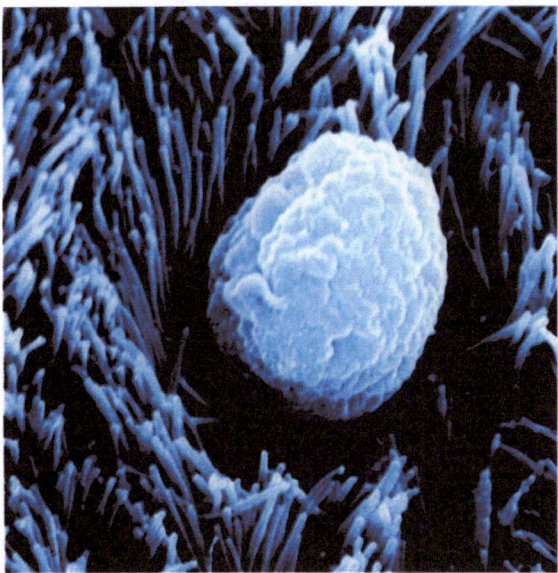

Fig. 3.1.e Main bronchus. Another goblet cell during the secretory process. Note the irregular surface, which permits the underlying granular structure of mucus which will be released to be appreciated (×5700)

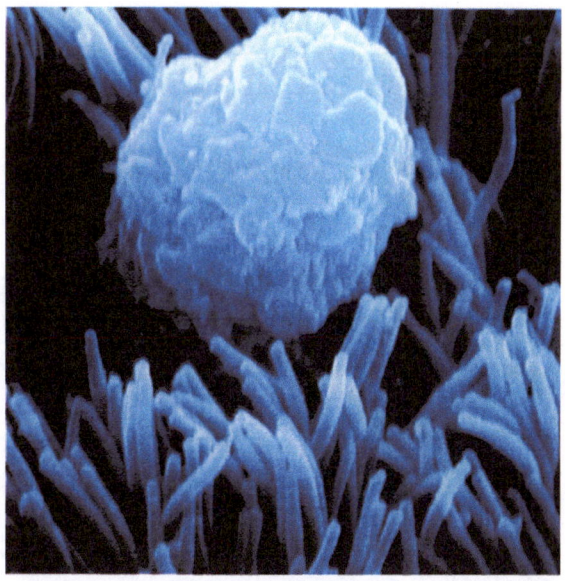

Fig. 3.1.f On this scanning electron micrograph at higher magnification (×6200), it is possible to see that the mucus secreting process is on its ultimate phase. The apical part of the goblet is protruding so much that it is lying over the tips of the cilia. The different globules of mucus and their outlines are clearly evident

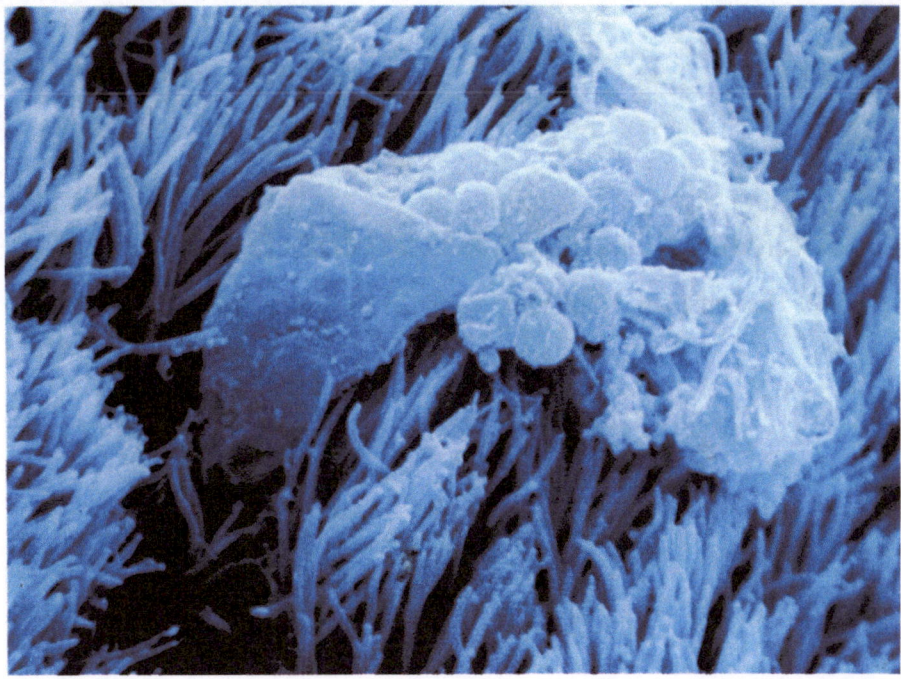

Fig. 3.2. Last step of the mucus secreting process. We can see a goblet cell with its body partially over the surrounding cilia releasing small globules of mucus over the cilia surface (×4580)

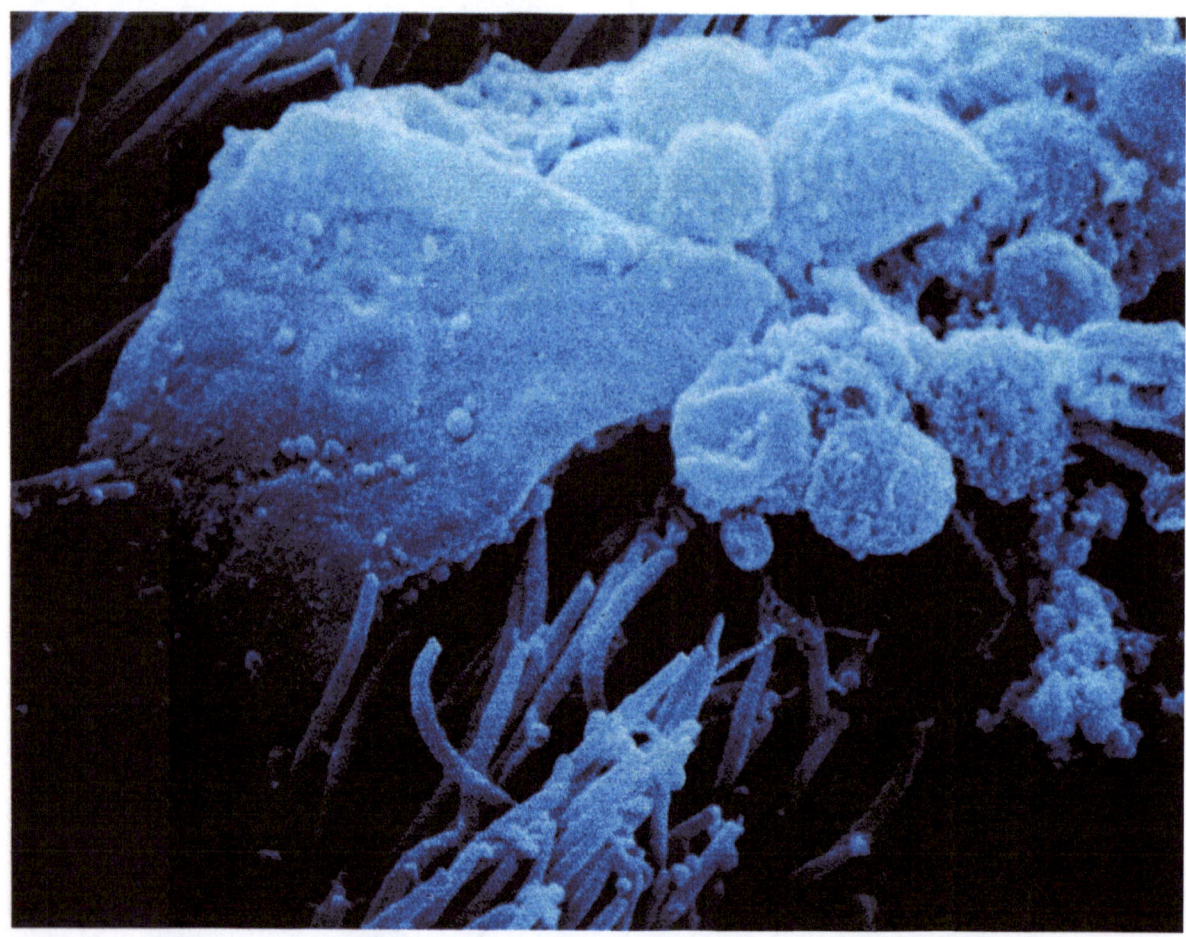

Fig. 3.3. The same area as in Fig. 3.2 seen at higher magnification (×9150)

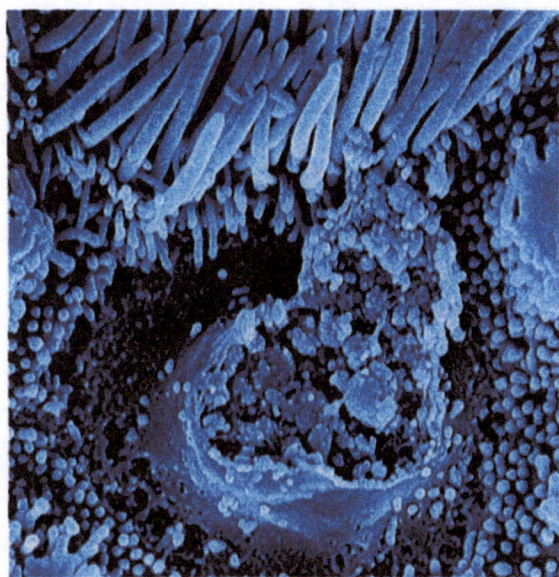

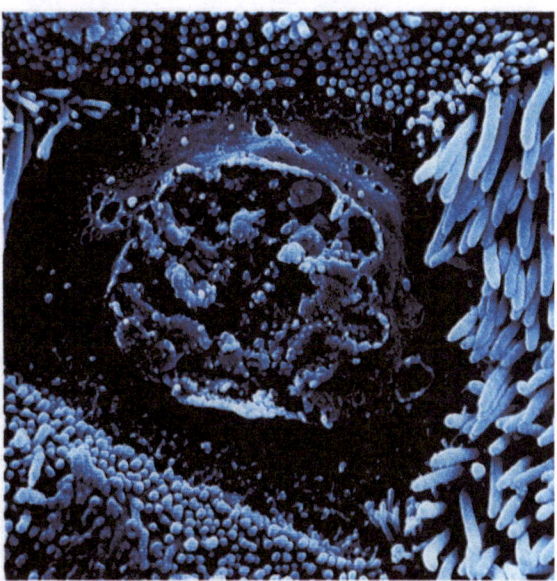

Fig. 3.4. Goblet cell. When the secretory products accumulate under the apical portion of the cell, the external surface, normally only slightly dome-shaped and with microvilli, tends to increase its curvature and thus reduces the presence of microvilli. In this micrograph it is possible to see the mucous granules inside the apical part of a goblet cell when the overlying cellular membrane is removed (×7700)

Fig. 3.5. Another goblet cell without its apical membrane showing the globules of mucus (×7050)

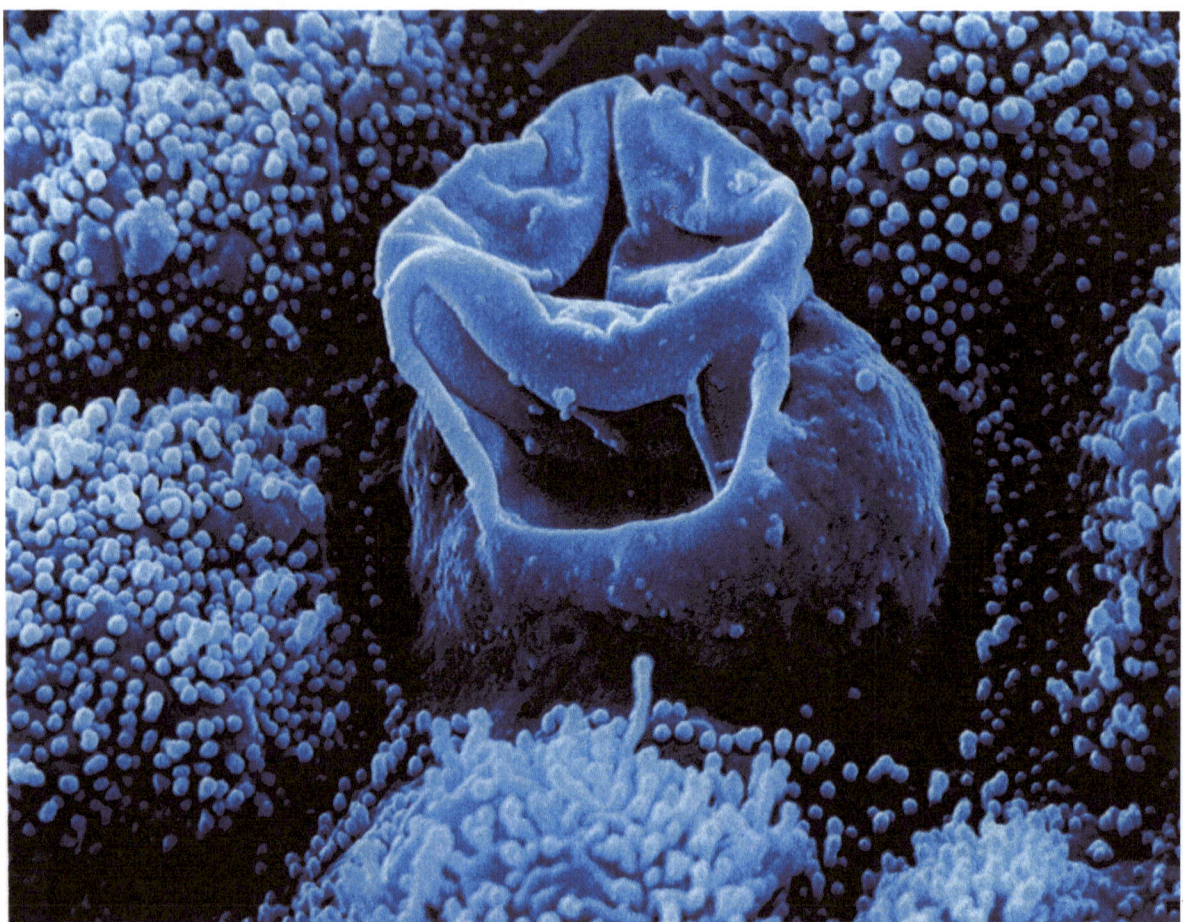

Fig. 3.6. When a goblet cell is empty of its secretory products it can sometimes collapse and assume the appearance of an empty bag (×6500). Around the empty goblet cell are other goblet cells with microvilli and at different stages of the mucus secreting process

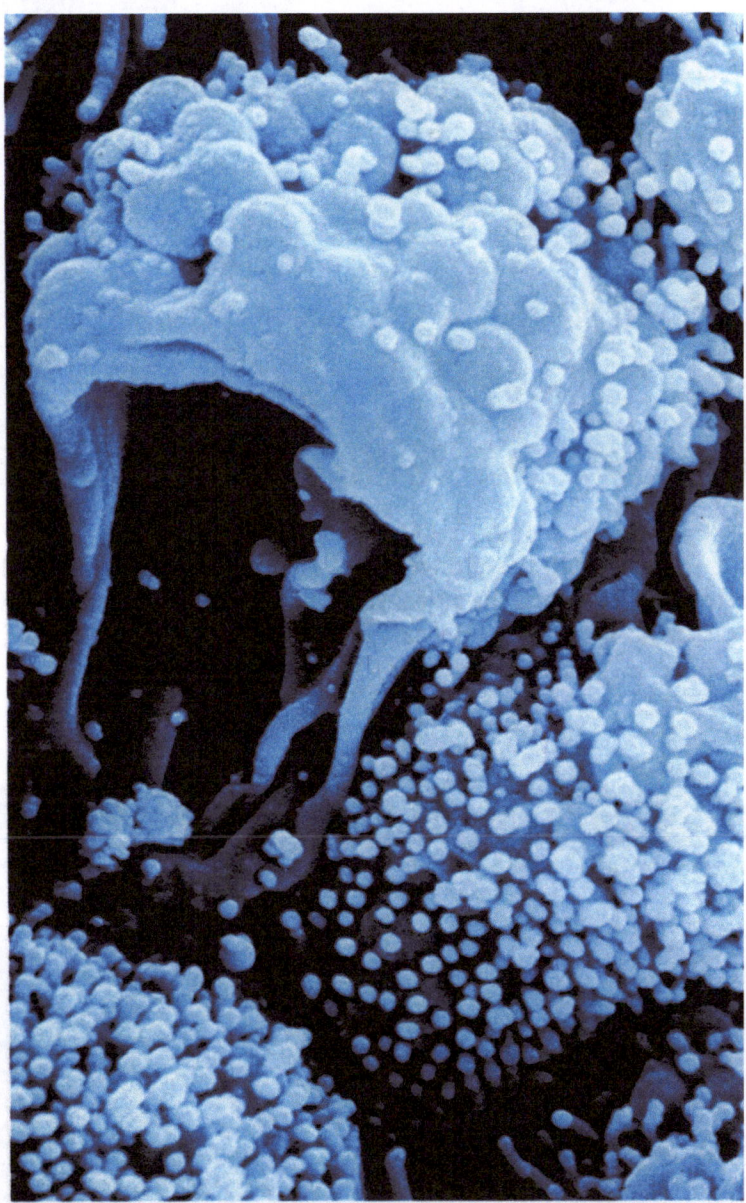

Fig. 3.7. Another view of an empty goblet cell (×10000)

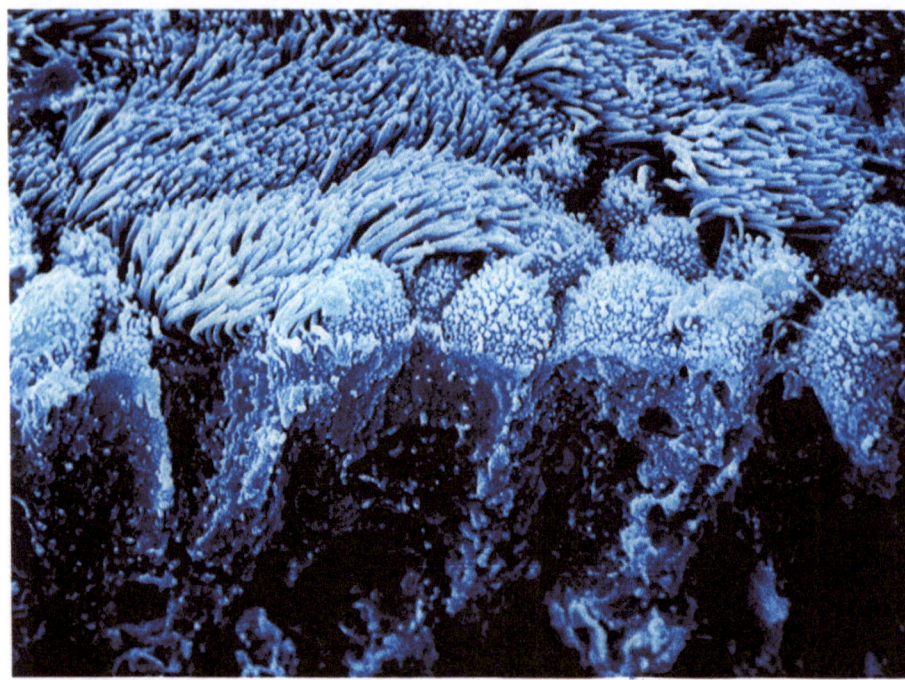

Fig. 3.8. Epithelial edge of the pseudostratified epithelium, obtained by freeze-fracture, showing both the surface and the lateral views of goblet cells. The dome-shaped structure of the apical part of the goblet cell is evident with the surface rich in microvilli and part of the cells under the plane of ciliary insertion (×2620)

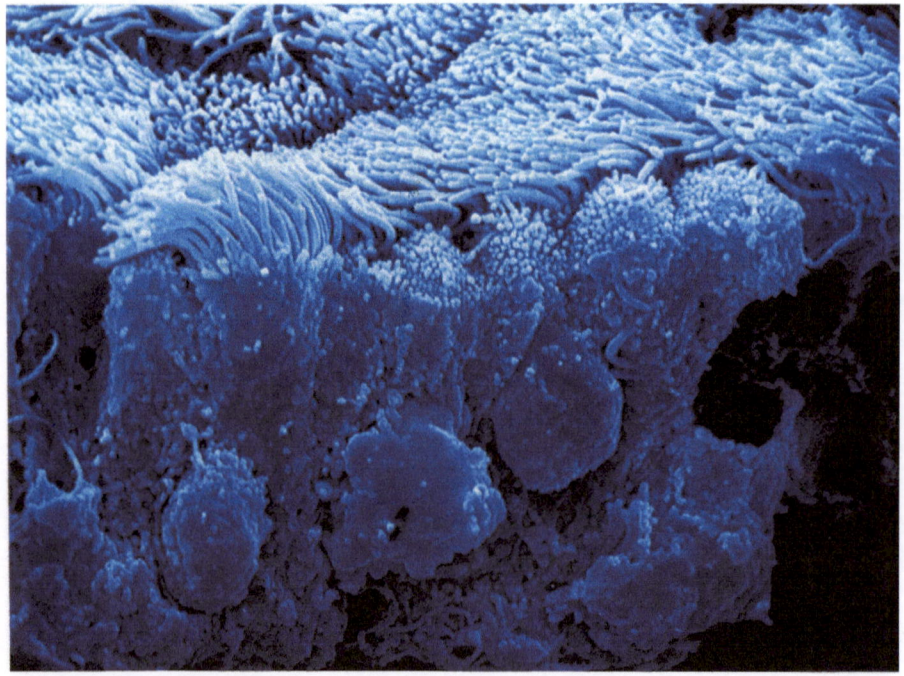

Fig. 3.9. The same view as in Fig. 3.8 with basal cells also present (×2720)

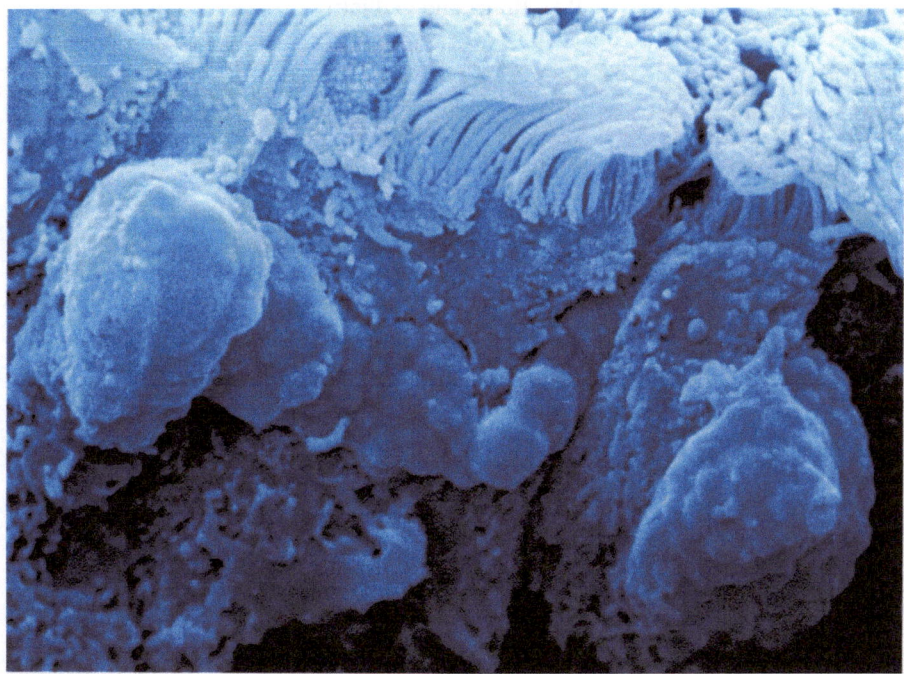

Fig. 3.10. Freeze-fracture of the epithelium of a bronchus. The globular structure of the goblet cells is evident. Under the membrane some small globules of secretions are visible (×3700)

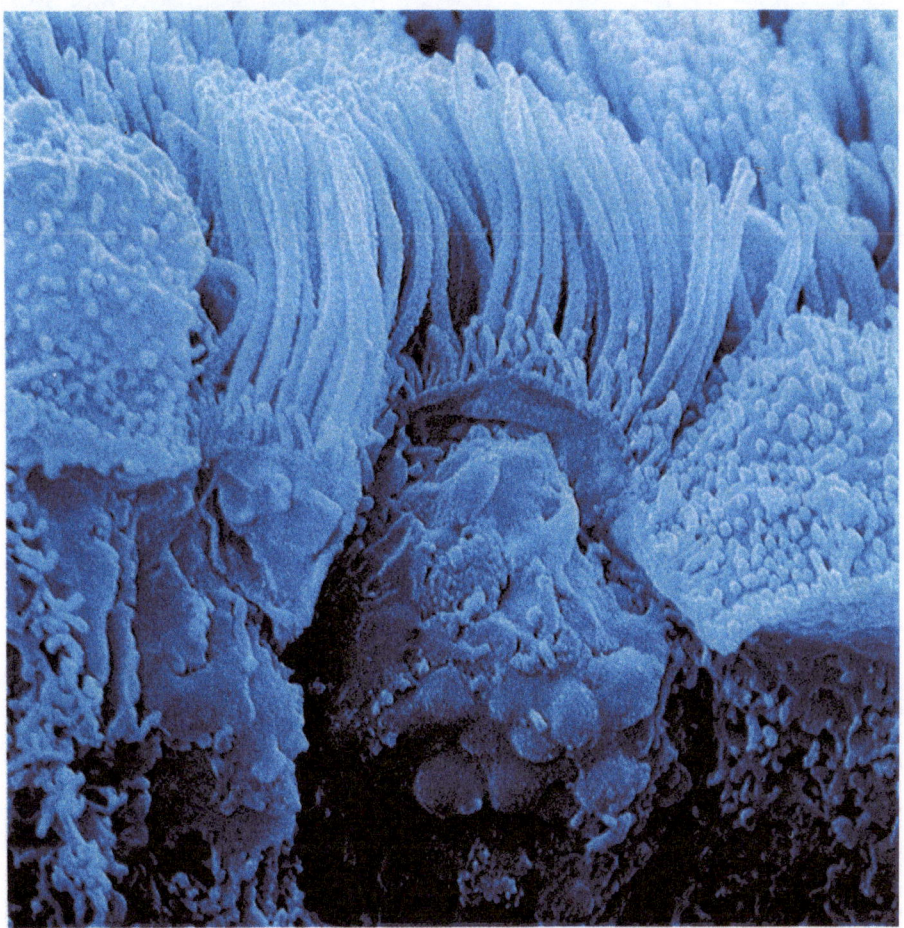

Fig. 3.11. Both ciliated cells with their microvilli and globules of secretions are clearly visible in the lower part of the central goblet cell (×5450)

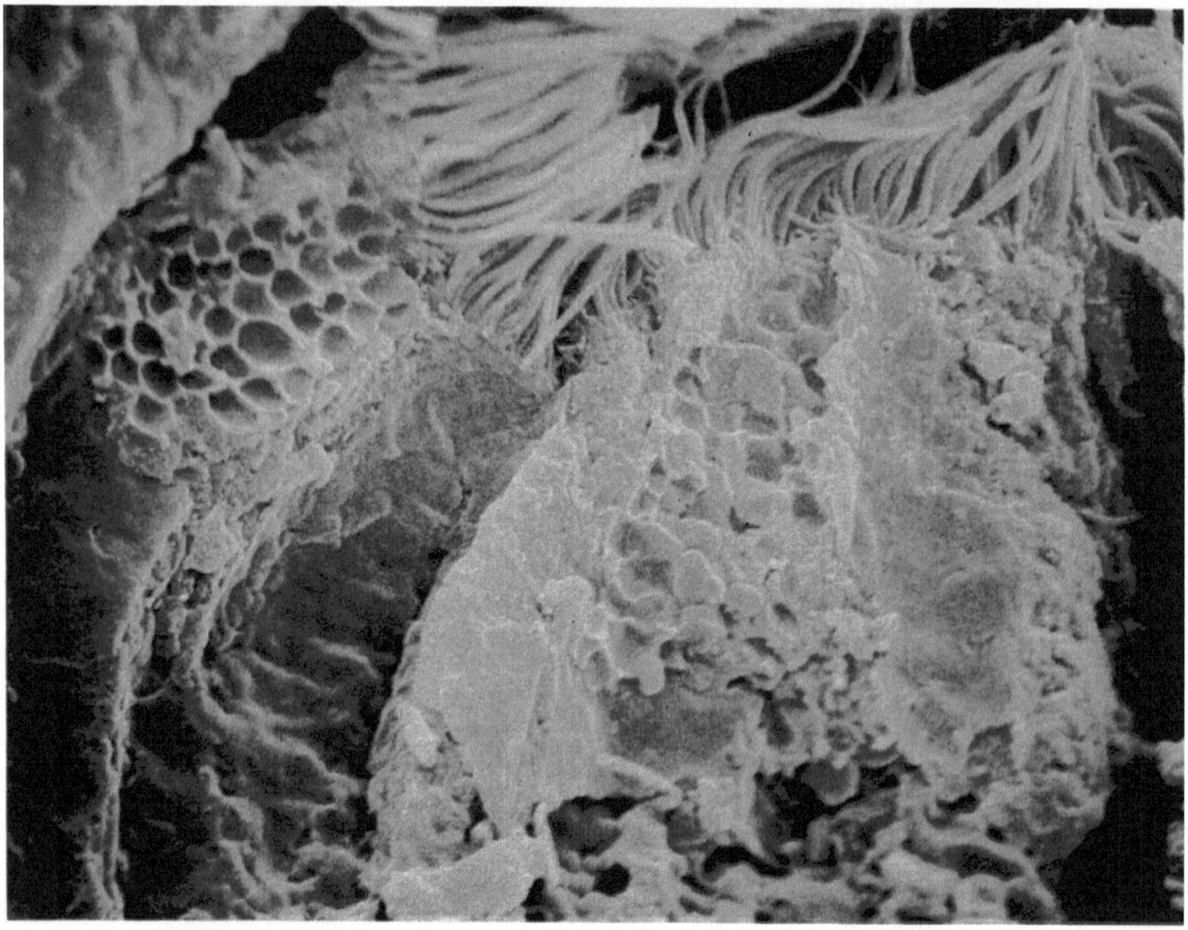

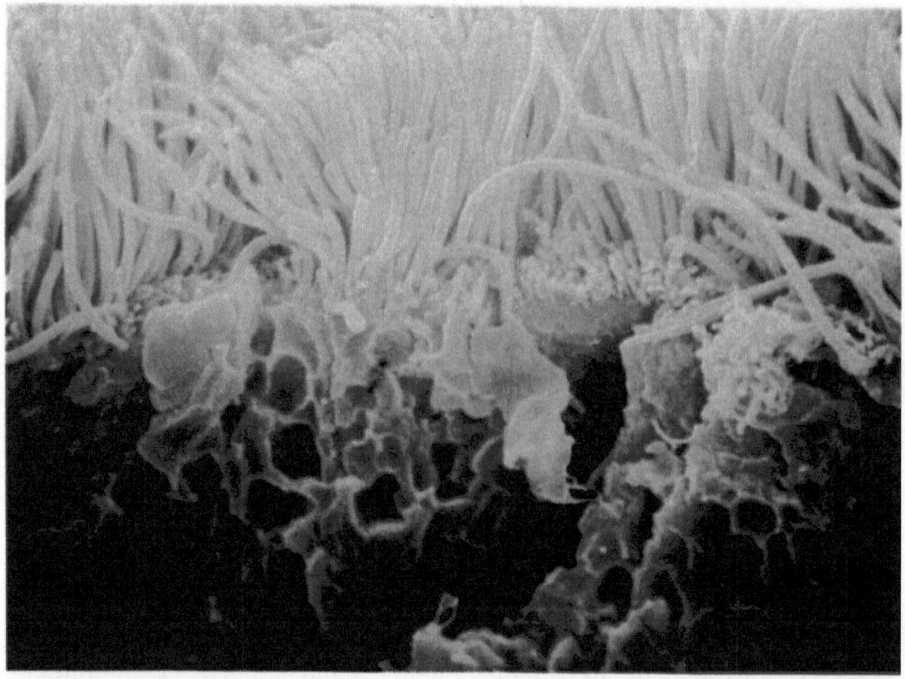

Fig. 3.12. In this freeze-fracture of the epithelium of a bronchus it is possible to see the internal architecture of two goblet cells. The small cavities are in some cases empty and in others still contain globules of secretion (×3240)

Fig. 3.13. Same situation as in Fig. 3.12 from another perspective (×5200)

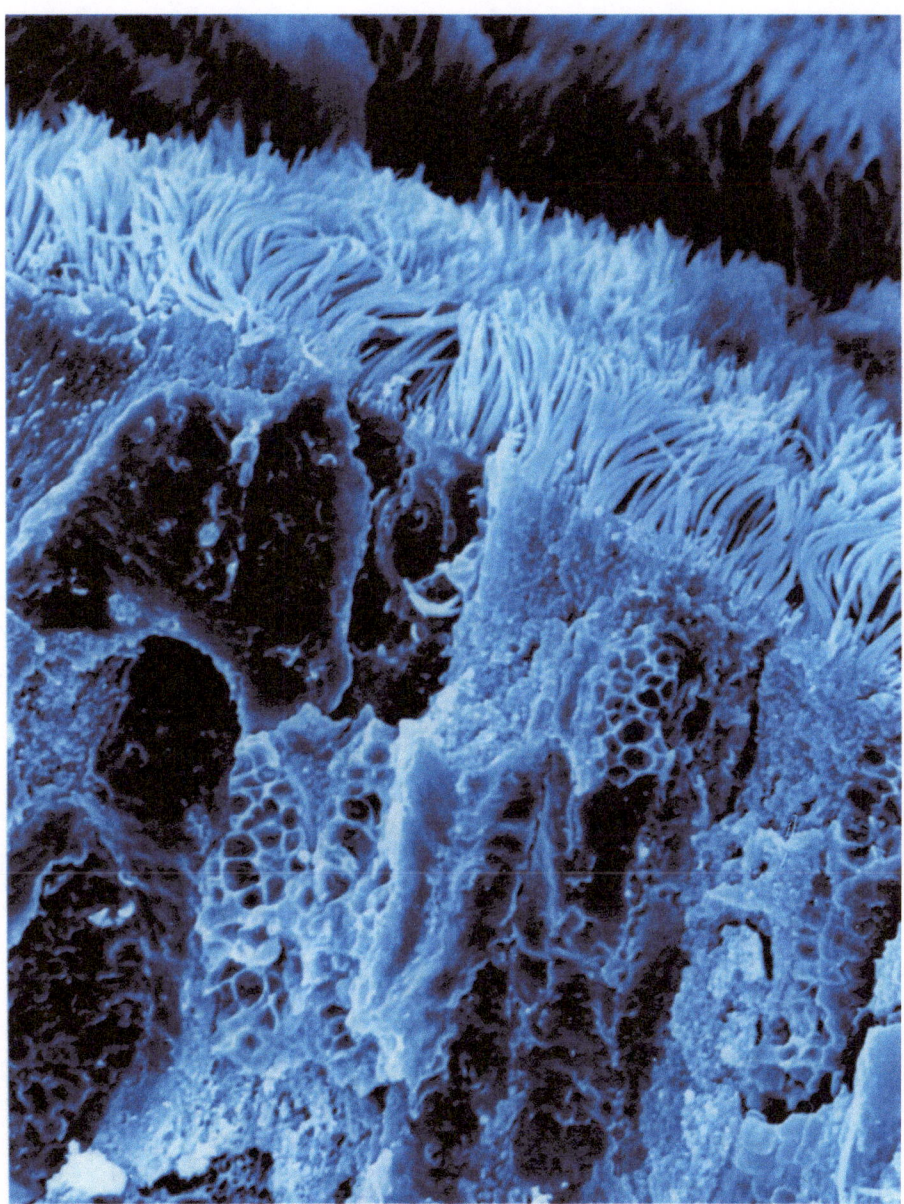

Fig. 3.14. A cut fracture of the epithelium of a bronchus showing, where the cell membrane has been broken, the hive structure of mucous globules of goblet cells (×3170)

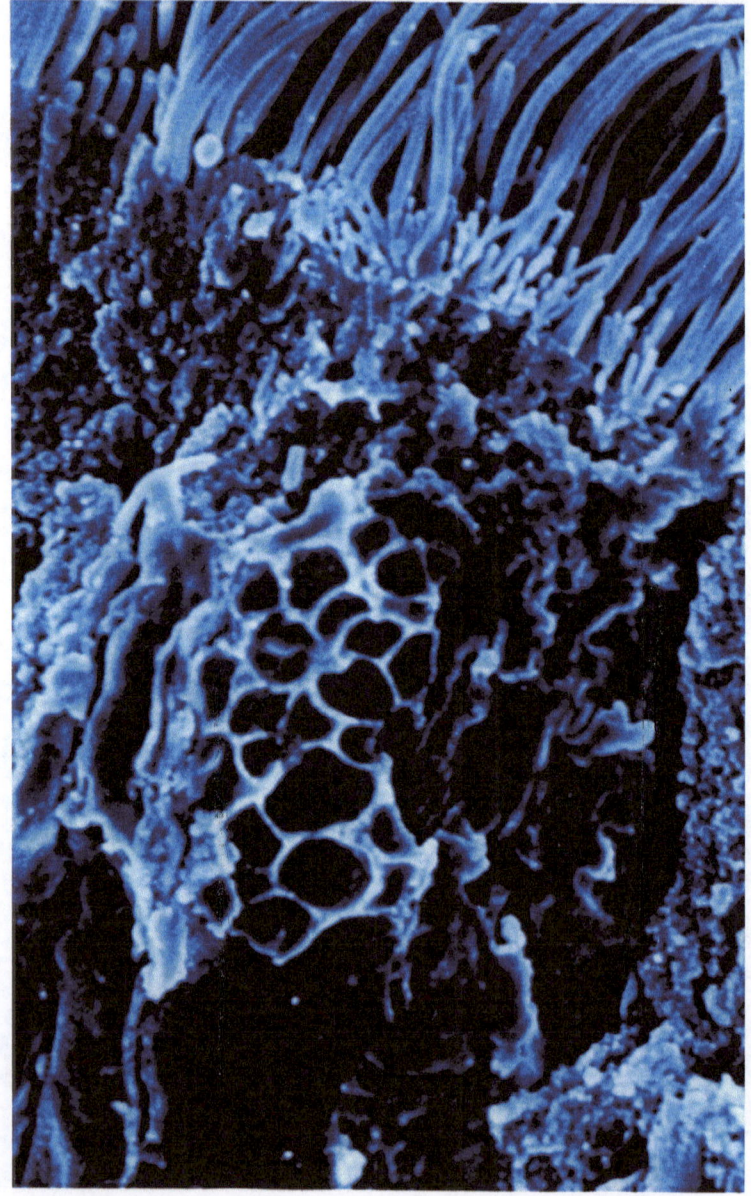

Fig. 3.15. Enlargement of a part of Fig. 3.14 (×4200)

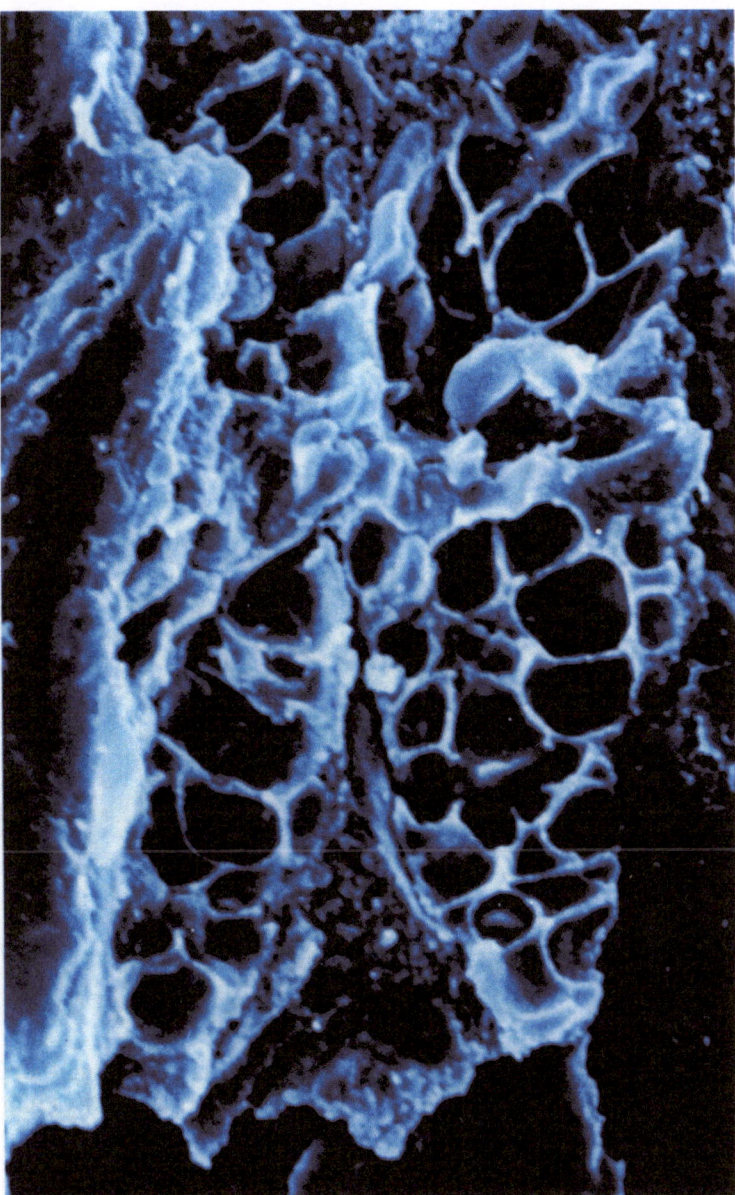

Fig. 3.16. With a further enlargement it is possible to see that the globules of secretion are separated each other by a thin membrane ($\times$5610)

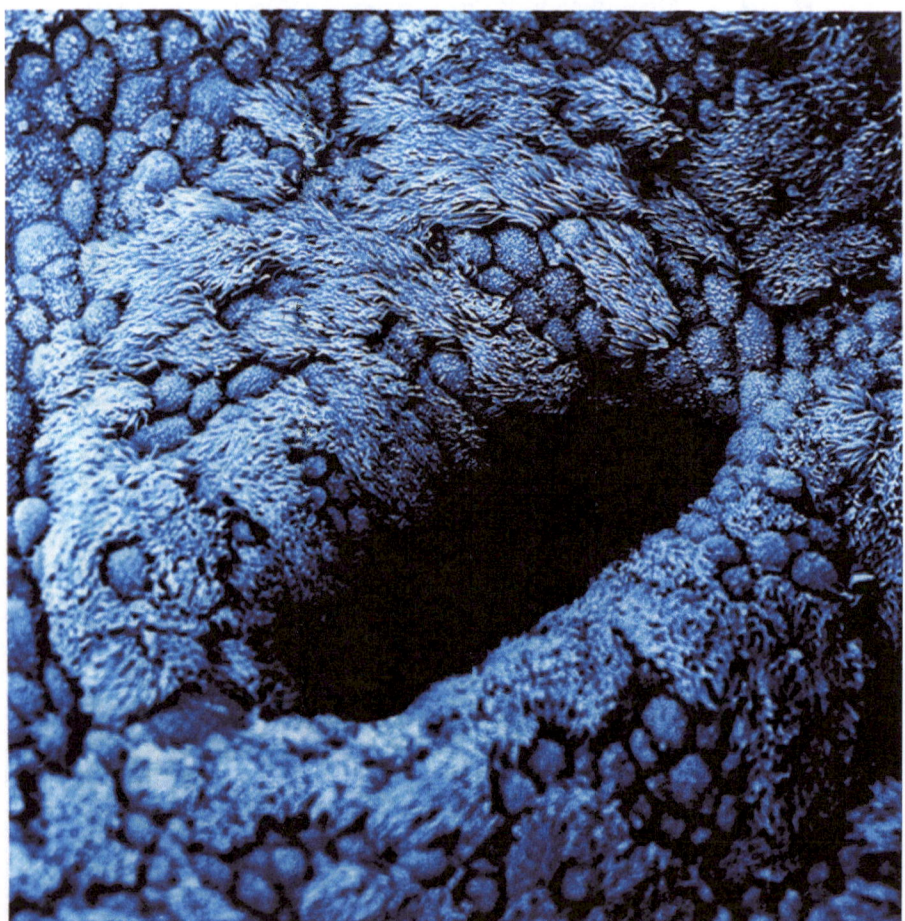

Fig. 3.17. Opening of a duct of a submucosal gland into the luminal surface of a bronchus. This opening appears as a "black hole" surrounded by ciliated cells (×680)

Chapter 4
Mucociliary Transport and SEM

P. C. Braga and G. Piatti

Centro di Farmacologia Respiratoria, Facoltà di Medicina e Chirurgia,
Università degli Studi di Milano

Trancheobronchial mucus is a non-Newtonian viscoelastic material, and it has been observed that changes in its chemical composition induce changes in its physical properties.

Mucus and moving cilia interact with each other, resulting, under physiological conditions, in a transport mechanism for mucus called "mucociliary clearance". This kind of transport is regulated by cohesive and adhesive forces.

Adhesion is a physical phenomenon involving forces between unlike molecules. In tracheobronchial mucus transport, it is involved in the frictional forces and in the reciprocal attractive physicochemical bonds at the interface between the gel phase and cilia (or airway surface). The significance of adhesiveness or adhesive forces in mucociliary clearance mechanism is not clear and its clinical and pharmacological aspects have not been extensively investigated.

Cohesion is a physical phenomenon involving forces between like molecules. In tracheobronchial mucus transport, it is involved in the crosslinking bonds among the macromolecules, ions, etc., inside the mucus, determining the so-called rheological properties of mucus (viscosity, elasticity).

Cilia supply the force which acts on mucus to move it. Acted upon by this force, mucus can either be deformed and/or flow. Rheology is the branch of physics that studies the deformation and flow of matter. The way the mucus responds to forces with deformation and/or flowing is the so-called rheological behavior of mucus. The forces exerted by the cilia act on the internal cohesion forces of mucus and on its rheological properties: viscosity and elasticity.

The mucus gel is an anisotropic polymeric viscoelastic material that behaves partially as a fluid and partially as a solid. As a fluid, mucus flows under forces applied by cilia, and this reveals its viscosity, which is a measure of the resistance (internal cohesion) of a fluid to flow. As a solid, mucus undergoes an elastic deformation under forces applied by cilia, and this reveals its elasticity, which is a measure of the capacity of a deformed material to return to its original shape. When forces (or energy) are applied to mucus, it stores part of this energy by elastic deformation; this energy is relased when the deforming force is removed, so mucus demonstrates elastic recovery.

Mucus is transported through alternating phases of flow (viscosity) and of elastic recovery (elasticity). It appears that good (relatively high) elastic recoil (stored energy) together with relatively low viscosity (resistance) are optimal rheological conditions for good mucociliary clearance.

Since cilia are beating during mucus transport, and mucus is flowing, SEM observations cannot give information about this phenomenon, because they are of necessity made on fixed material under vacuum. Nevertheless, SEM observations are very important, because in a sample of trachea or bronchial ciliated epithelium observed by SEM, the different steps of ciliary movement are "frozen" and so one can observe the mechanics of this phenomenon. Moreover, the different relationships between mucus cilia and the periciliary layer can be observed in a fascinating tridimensional picture.

Mucociliary transport is necessary to maintain both the physiological function of the respiratory apparatus and health. SEM images clearly support the idea that mucus is transported by the tips of the cilia, which penetrate the lower surface of the mucus during their effective stroke. If the periciliary layer is too thick, the cilia cannot come into contact with mucus, and propulsion will be ineffective. It will also be ineffective if the periciliary layer is too shallow, in which situation the cilia come too strongly into contact with mucus, preventing them from completing their beat cycle.

Acknowledgements. The authors thank Raven Press, New York, for permission to reproduce the micrograph in Fig. 4.11, from Guffanti EE, Vercelloni SM, Piatti G, Braga PC (1990) Cilia and mucociliary clearance. In: Allegra L, Braga PC (eds) Bronchial Mucology and related diseases. Raven Press, New York, p. 36.

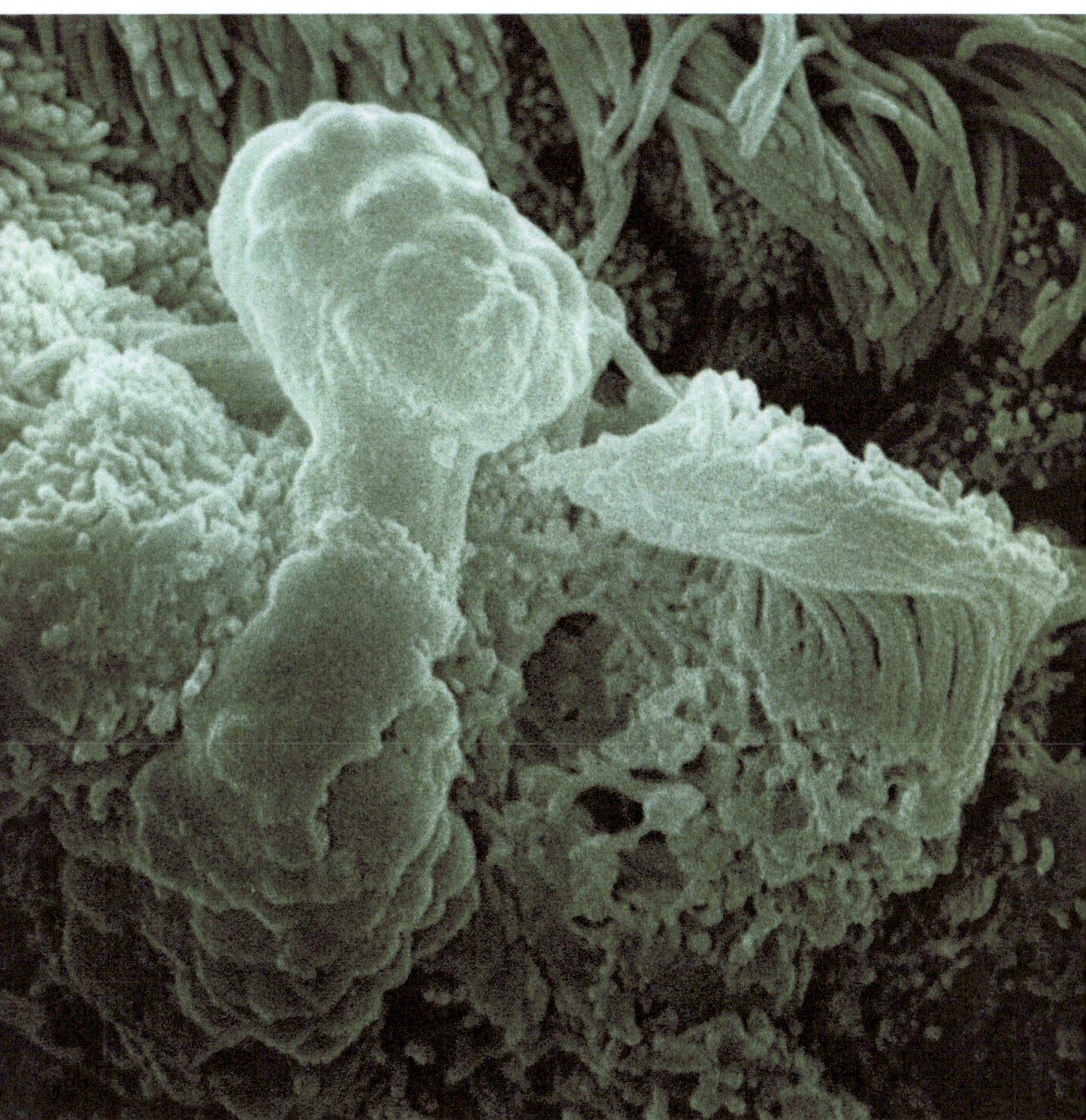

Fig. 4.1. Freeze-fracture of a specimen of trachea, showing the epithelial edge. This picture is very interesting because it provides not only morphological but also functional information. Luck enabled the moment to be frozen when a goblet cell, whose characteristic body with its glomerular aspect is below the imaginary line of the epithelial margin, released a cloud of secretion over the imaginary line of the epithelial margin, while near it there is a bundle of cilia which seems to be waiting to transport the mucus (×5200)

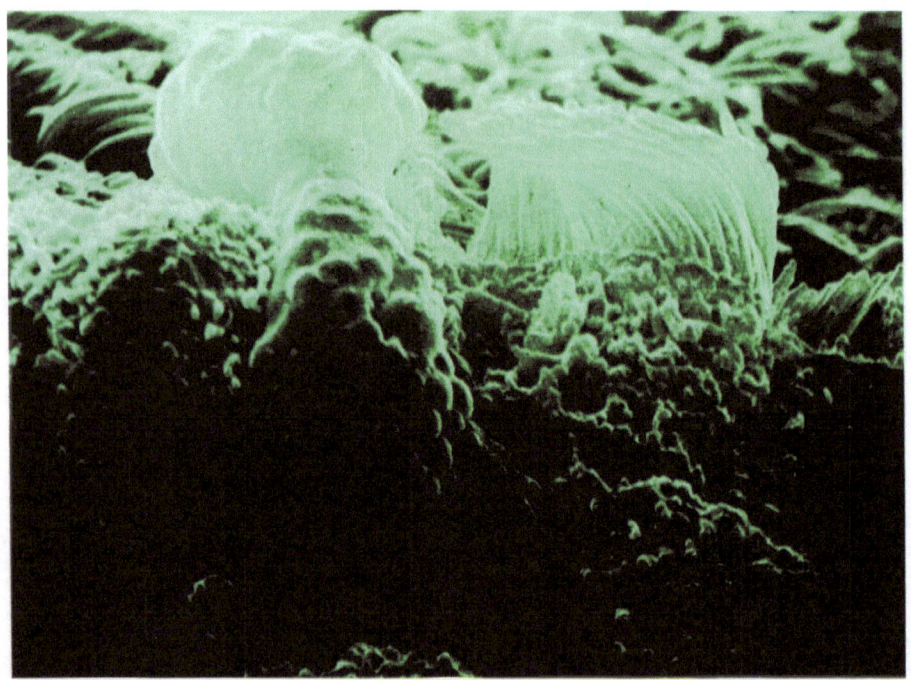

Fig. 4.2. The same freeze-fracture as in Fig. 4.1, but seen from another point of view (from below) (×5000). Morphofunctional aspects are clearly appreciated even at this point of view

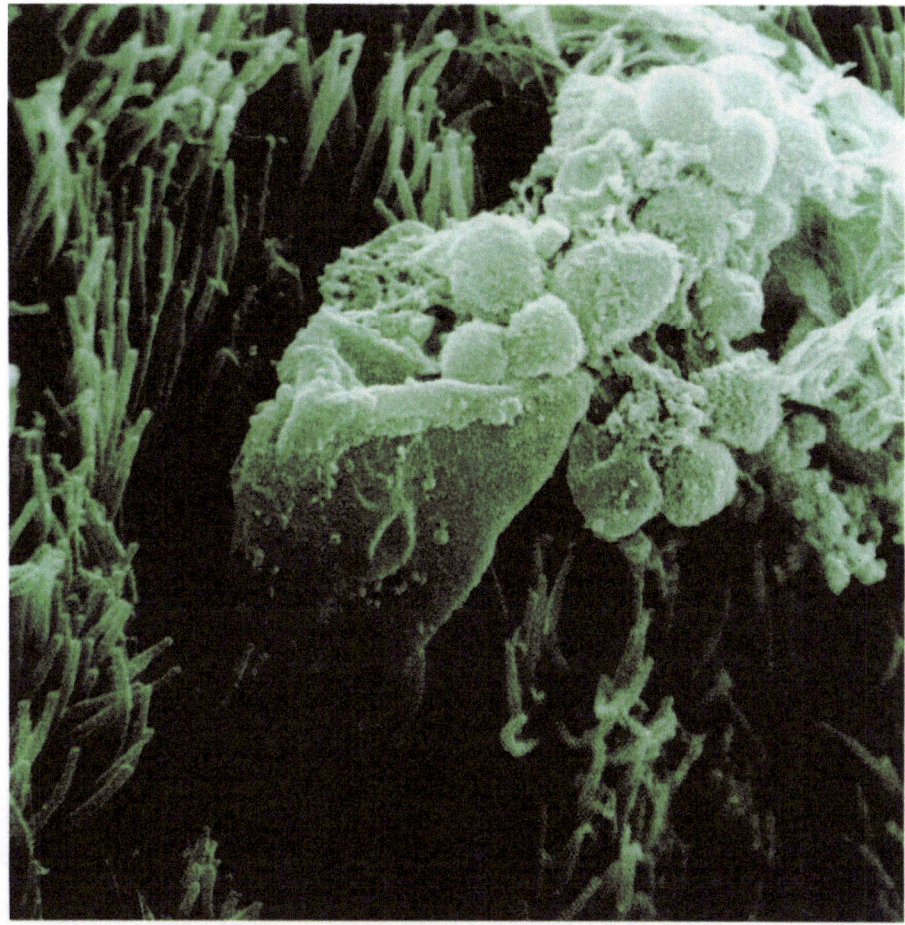

Fig. 4.3. After the rupture of the membrane of the apical part of a goblet cell, the granules of secretory product drop onto the tips of the cilia and spread along the ciliary carpet (×5000)

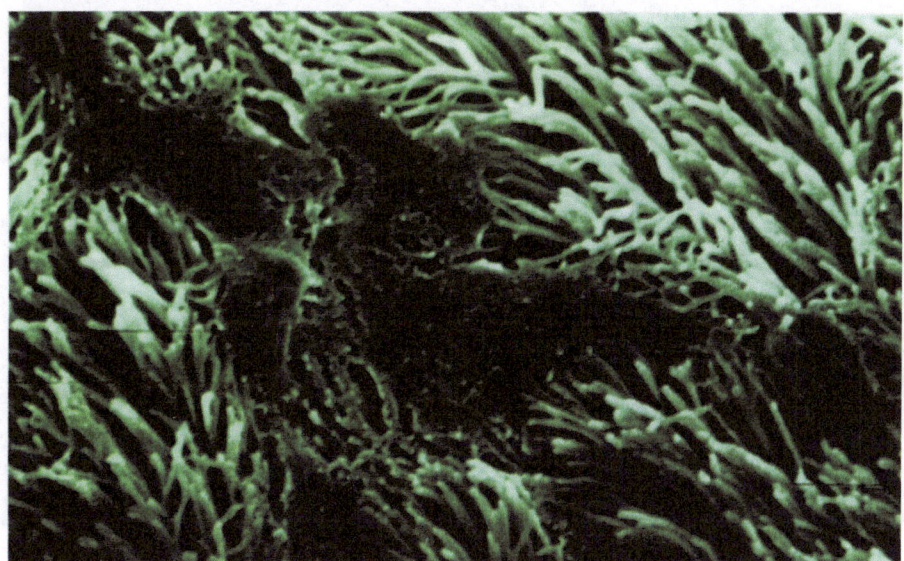

Fig. 4.4. The movement of the cilia spread the contents of the globules in an initially small smooth sheet of mucus (×2500)

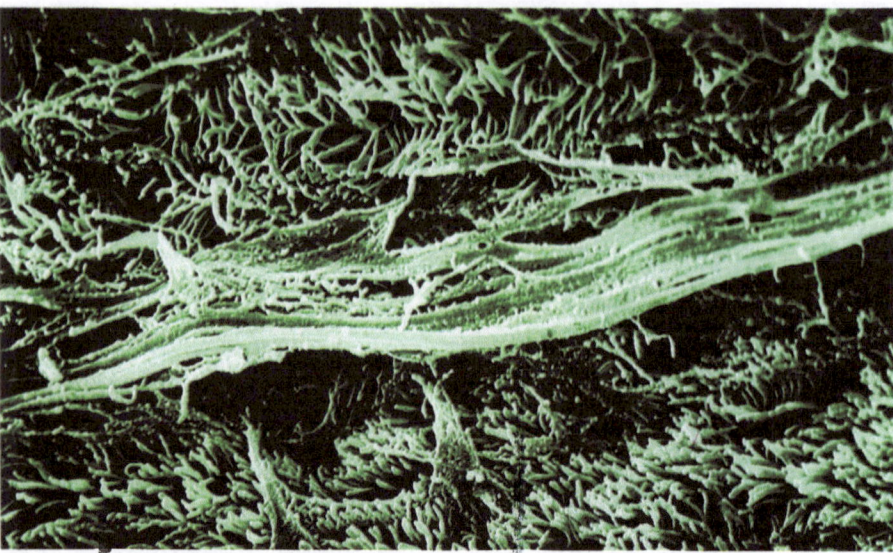

Fig. 4.5. The continous oscillatory movements of the cilia mobilize the small mucous sheets, thus forming a mucous blanket, with fibrillar aspect (×1930)

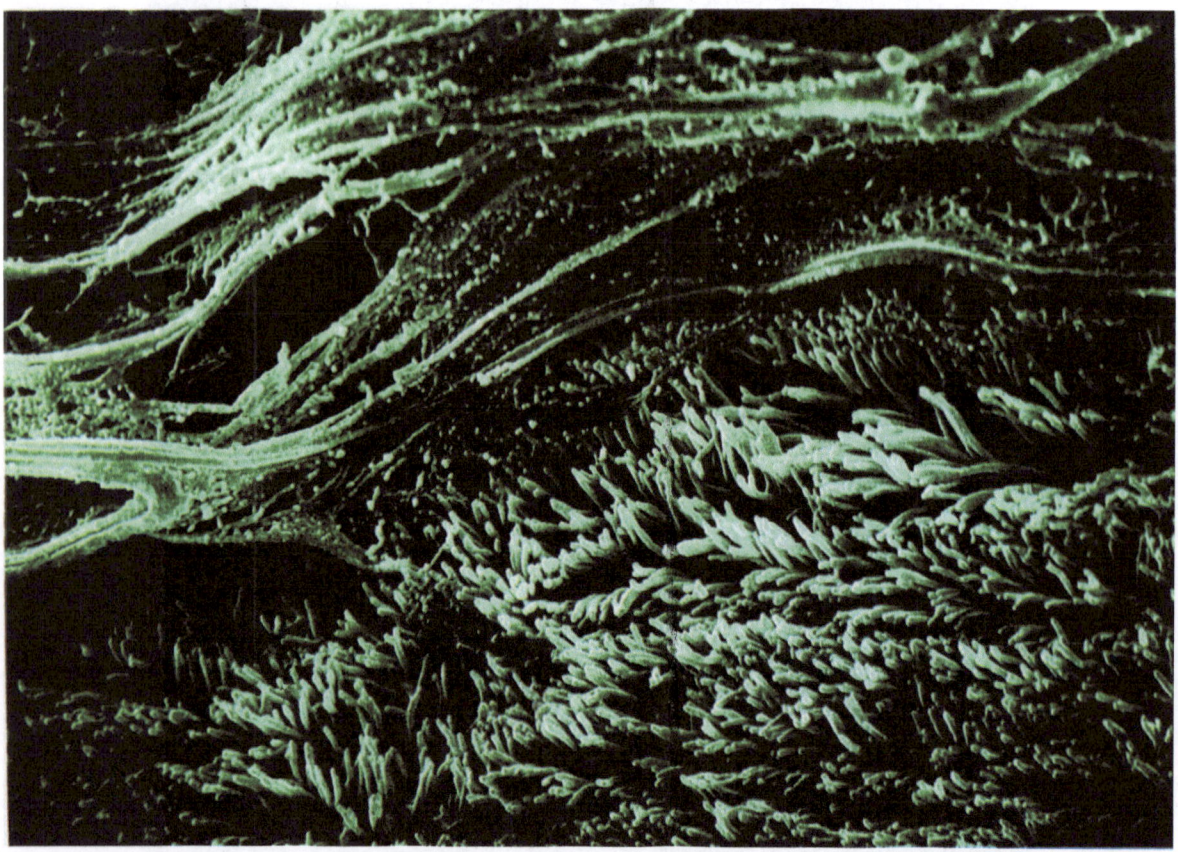

Fig. 4.6. Fig. 4.6. Mucus forming a blanket lying over the tips of the ciliated epithelium (×2400)

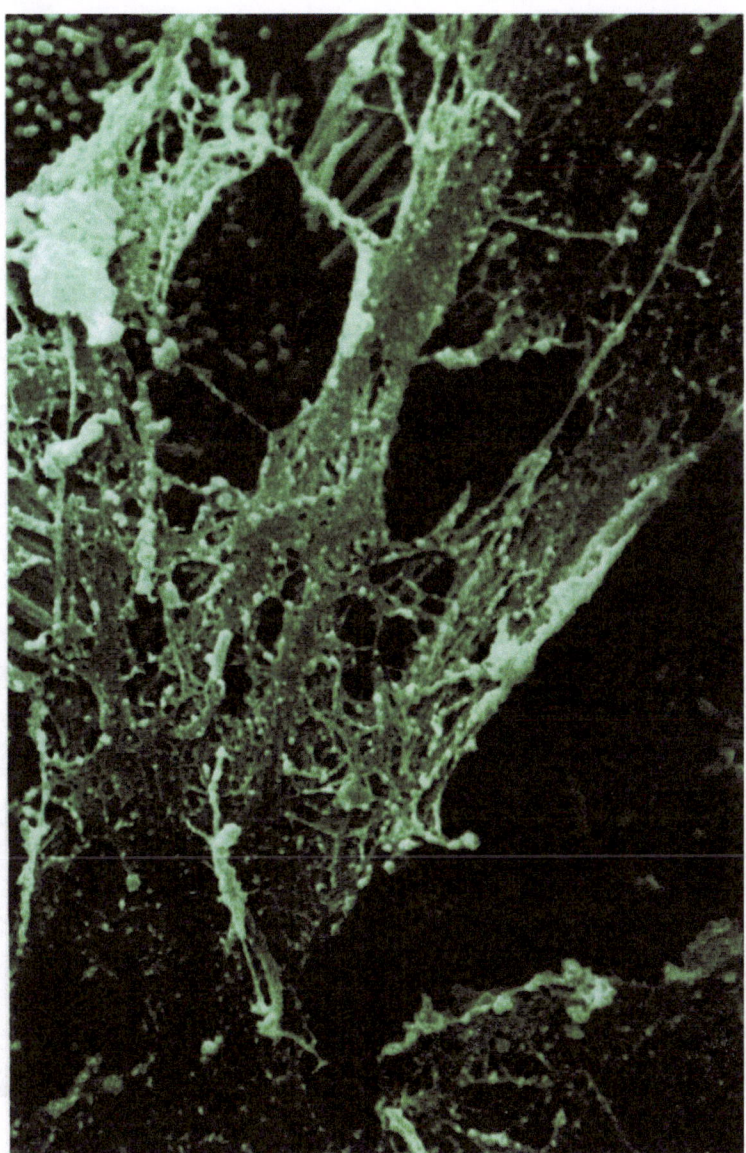

Fig. 4.7. Another view, from above of the cohesive mucous sheet that covers the underlying epithelium. Under the sheet are visible goblet and ciliated cells (×2500)

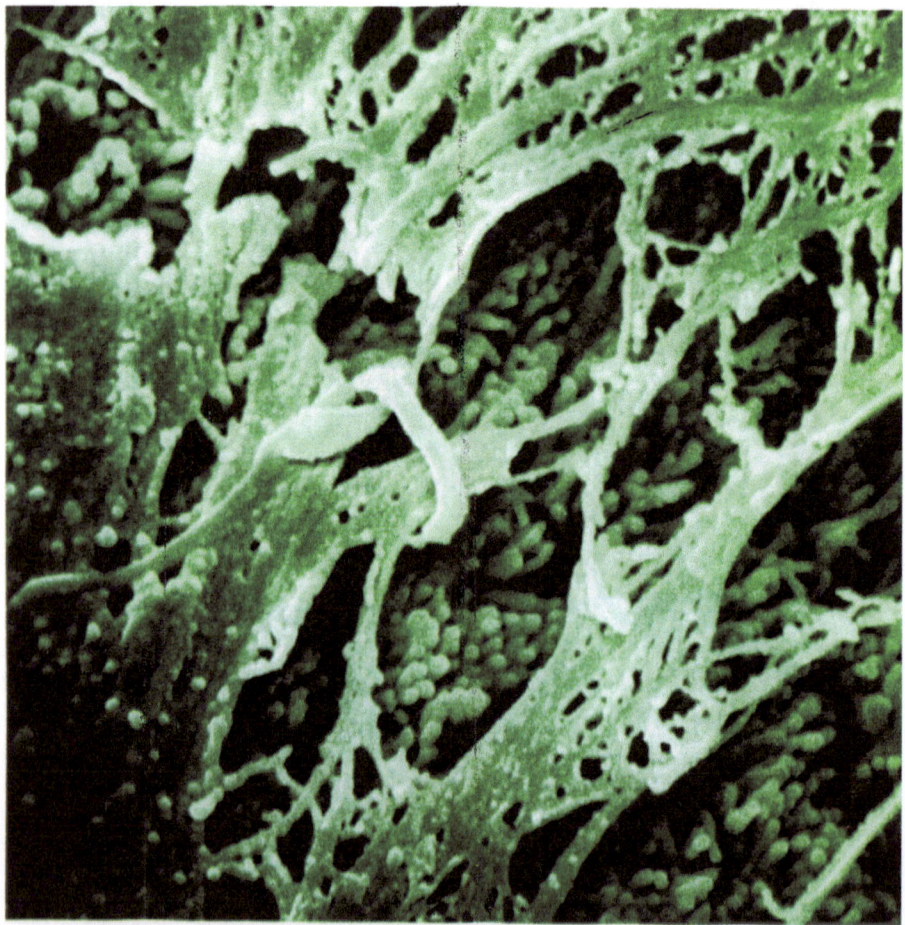

Fig. 4.8. The mucous sheet is a continuum at some points while at some other points it assumes a filamentous aspect (×2300)

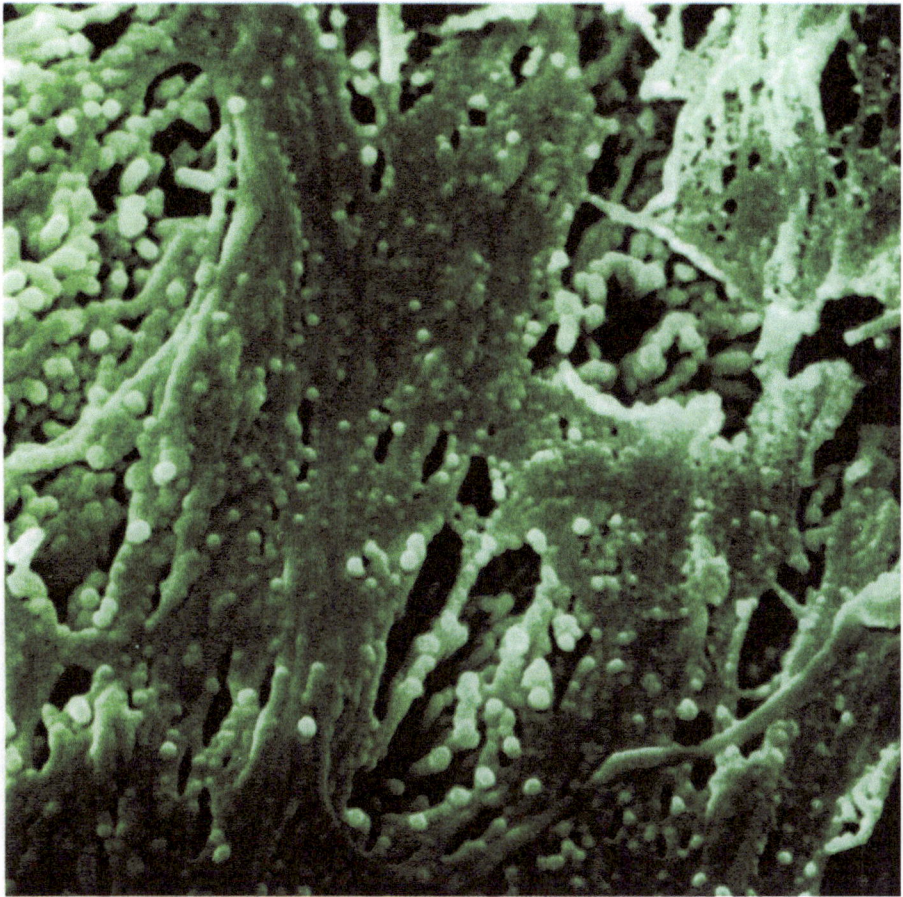

Fig. 4.9. In this micrograph it is interesting to observe the mucous sheet covering the cilia. The small white dots on the sheet are the tips of cilia which, for proper mucociliary clearance, must enter the sheet only for about 5000–9000 Å (×2300)

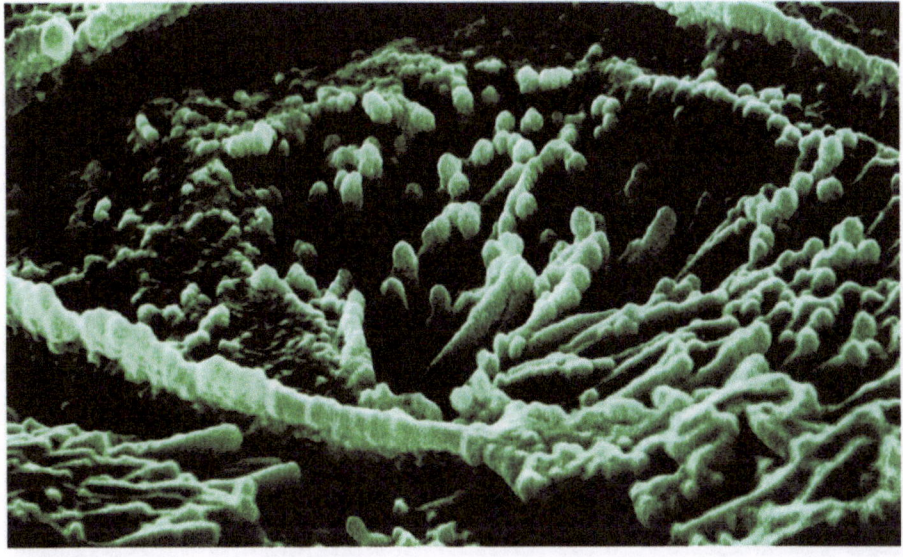

Fig. 4.10. The mucous blanket is sometimes interrupted by small holes in which are visible the tips of the underlying cilia (×9150)

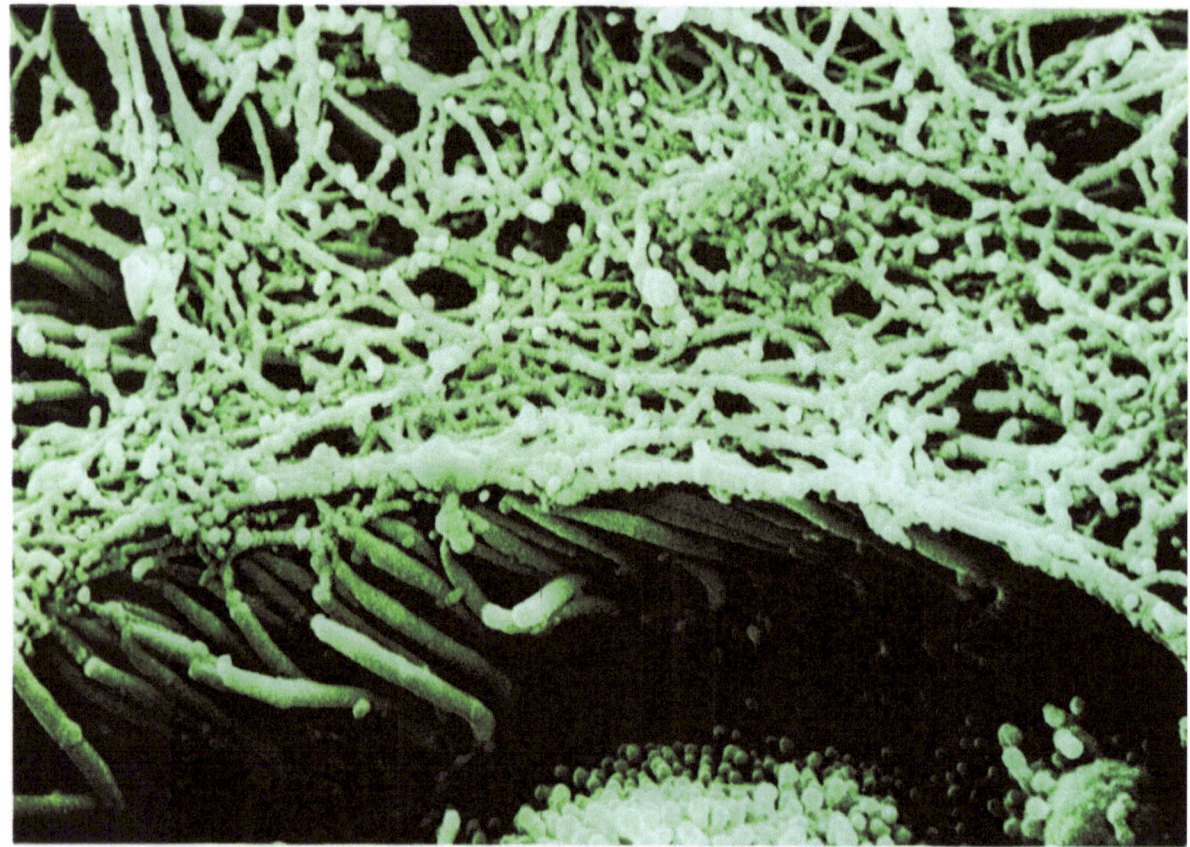

Fig. 4.11. This is another very interesting morphofunctional image which shows how mucociliary clearance happens. In the *upper part,* the mucous sheet with its fibrillar network is clearly evident, while in the *lower part* the cilia underlying the mucous sheet can be seen, only their tips making contact with the mucus. Some cilia are rigid (active phase) while others are bending to different degrees (recovery phase) ($\times 7700$)

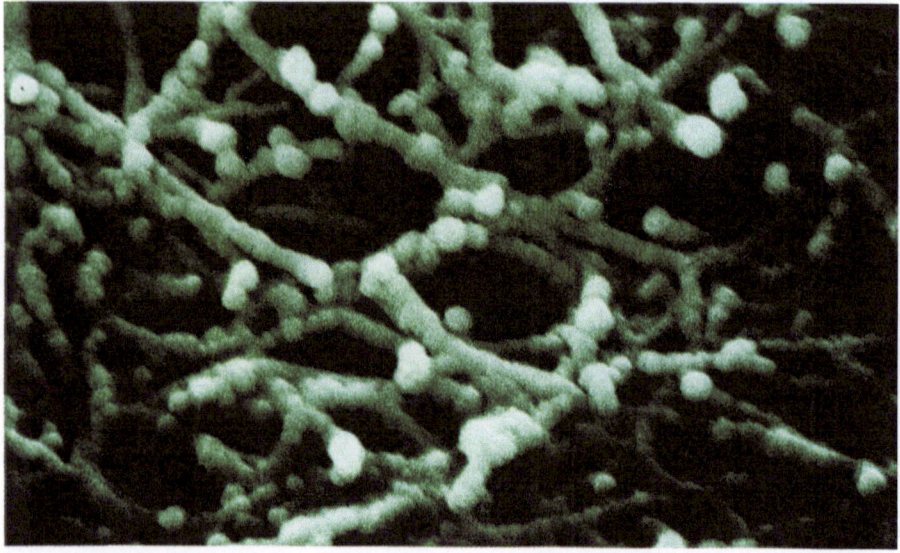

Fig. 4.12. Reticular and fibrillar network of the mucous layer at high magnification ($\times 24800$)

Chapter 5
Bronchioli as Visualized by SEM

L. Allegra and G. Piatti*

Istituto di Malattie Respiratorie, Facoltà di Medicina e Chirurgia,
Università degli Studi di Milano

*Centro di Farmacologia Respiratoria, Facoltà di Medicina e Chirurgia,
Università degli Studi di Milano

Bronchioles are intrapulmonary airways that start from the 4th generation and continuously bifurcate until they reach the alveolar ducts. They are called terminal bronchioles from the 15th to the 16th generations and respiratory bronchioles from the 17th to the 19th generation [1]. The caliber of the airways decreases from the trachea to the distal branches: bronchioles are approximately 1 mm in diameter or less. While surprisingly numerous, they are very short in length [2, 3].

The walls of these small conducting airways have the same basic structure as the large airways, being composed of a mucosa, a submucosa, and a fibrous layer, but there are some differences. The cartilage rings of the major bronchi are replaced by cartilage plates and more distally, in the terminal bronchioles, cartilage is completely absent. As the amount of cartilage decreases, elastic and muscular components increase and the bronchiolar wall becomes more flexible. The whole bronchial tree can thus change in volume in relation to the phase and intensity of respiration.

The smooth muscle bundles that form a continuous sleeve in the connective tissue underlying the epithelium are first circular and then spiral; their contraction narrows the lumen and shortens the length of the airways. A contraction of the smooth muscle in the bronchial wall produces a "corrugated" appearance of the mucosa, sometimes visible by SEM in cross sections. Bronchial glands are usually present in the submucosa of cartilaginous bronchi, but are not found in the membranous bronchioles.

The airway epithelium also changes progressively from the large bronchi to the bronchioles to the alveolar region. As can be appreciated by SEM, the pseudostratified type in the large airways becomes monostratified more peripherally, so that the bronchioles are lined with simple low columnar or cuboidal cells overlying the thin basal membrane [4].

While the larger bronchioles may have some microvilli-covered goblet cells intermingled with ciliated cells, there are none in the smaller bronchioles. Ciliated cells continue to the terminal bronchioles and sometimes to the proximal portion of the respiratory bronchioles, although their numbers decrease and the cilia are typically shorter (3–4 μm) than those found on the taller columnar cells that line the bronchi [5].

At lower magnification, the surface of the small bronchiole appears "pebbly". At higher magnification, ciliated and non ciliated areas are easily visible, the cilia having the appearance of bushes scattered over a field [6]. Each ciliated cell at this level has no more than 50 cilia.

A new cell type characterizes the bronchiolar wall: these so-called Clara cells are easily discerned by SEM since they protrudes considerably into the lumen. The ratio of ciliated to Clara cells changes proceeding peripherally toward the respiratory bronchioles, Clara cells becoming more common. The apex of a Clara cell shows a domed or papillary swelling which possesses a few microvilli and bulges markedly into the bronchiolar lumen.

The surface topography revealed by SEM is very impressive, and SEM continues to be of great value in understanding the microarchitecture of the bronchial wall at different levels of the airways. Although the functional significance of

Clara cells is subject to speculation, they are classified as active secretory cells because of their content of cell organelles and secretory granules, and it seems that may produce a component of the surfactant present in the alveoli [7].

Ultrastructural studies have been carried out in the mouse, the rat [8], the rabbit, the pig [9], the macaque [10], and man. Hypothesized roles of Clara cells include secretion of substances that modulate airway smooth muscle tone or liquid clearance and detoxification of inhaled agents. These cells release their secretory granules into the bronchiolar lumen by apocrine or/and neurocrine secretion. Their club-shaped apices may be more or less prominent, probably reflecting differences in the secretory phases or cell maturation. When the cell dome matures, it breaks up by dissolution of the cell membrane, and the released components mix themselves with the lining of the bronchiole surface. Clara cells synthesize the serous secretion which intermingles in the higher airways with the mucous layer of bronchial secretions [11]. In the respiratory bronchioles the number of Clara cells is considerably smaller and ciliated cells can only occasionally be observed.

In the distal portion of the respiratory bronchioles the wall abruptly becomes alveolarized, and the cuboidal epithelium becomes flattened and partially replaced by squamous epithelium (type I cells), essentially interfacing with the pneumocytes of the alveolar duct [12]. Small muscle and elastic bundles surround the point of passage from the bronchiolar wall to alveoli and form a sleeve that regulates air flow into alveoli.

When lungs are fixed by vascular perfusion it is possible to preserve the extracellular fluid that lines the bronchioles: in this situation the bronchiolar surface appears smooth, and cilia and Clara cells are embedded in an amorphous material which sits directly on the alveolar lining layer. The material is probably of mixed origin, coming from the Clara cells and the alveolar surface. This "bronchiolar surfactant" is important for ensuring bronchiolar stability during changes of pressure in the lung [13, 14].

The distal airways, and especially the respiratory bronchioles, are often the primary sites of effects due to by infectious agents and inhaled toxic irritants and it is therefore at this level that the first pathological alterations occur [15–17].

Every terminal bronchiole divides into two respiratory bronchioles, which in turn divide into 2–10 alveolar ducts; these terminal airways have a wall that is uninterrupted by alveoli. When observed with the SEM, the progression from terminal to respiratory bronchiole shows gradual change from a roughened luminal surface to a smooth surfaced epithelium. The beginning of the respiratory bronchiole is delineated from the terminal bronchiole proper by the presence of a few alveoli along the bronchiolar wall.

References

1. Fishman AP (1980) Pulmonary disease and disorders, vol 1. McGraw-Hill, New York, pp 11–44
2. Kessel RG, Kardon RH (1979) Tissue and organs: a text-atlas of SEM. Freeman, San Francisco, pp 203–217
3. Staub NC, Albertine KH (1988) The structure of the lungs relative to their principal function. In: Murray H, Nadel J (eds) Textbook of respiratory medicine. Saunders, London, pp 12–46
4. Andrews PM (1974) A scanning electron microscopic study of extrapulmonary respiratory tract. Am J Anat 139:399–424
5. Andrews PM (1979) The respiratory system. In: Hodges GH, Hallowes RC (eds) Biomedical research application of SEM. Academic, London, pp 177–202
6. Nai San Wang (1970) Scanning electron microscopy of the lung. Hum Pathol 1:227–231
7. St George JA, Harkema JR, Hyde DM, Plopper CG (1988) Cell populations and structure-function relationships of cells in the airways. In: Gardner DE, Crapo JD, Massaro EJ (eds) Toxicology of the lung. Raven, New York, pp 71–102
8. Souma T (1987) The distribution and surface ultrastructure of airway epithelial cells in the rat lung: a scanning electron microscopic study. Arch Histol Jap 50:419–436
9. Plopper CG, Mariassy AT, Hill LH (1980) Ultrastructure epithelial (Clara) cell of mammalian lung. II. A comparison of horse, steer, sheep, dog, cat. Exp Lung Res 1:155–169
10. Castleman WL, Dungworth DL, Tyler WS (1975) Intrapulmonary airway morphology in three species of monkeys: a correlated scanning and transmission electron microscopic study. Am J Anat 142:107–122
11. Roth J, Meyer HW (1972) Electron microscopic studies in mammalian lungs by freeze-etching. III. The bronchiolar cells with special consideration of the Clara cells. Exp Pathol 7:71–83

12. Davis ML, Lewandowski J, Dodson RF (1984) Morphology and ultrastructure of the distal airway epithelium in the guinea pig. Anat Rec 209:509–522

13. Gil J, Weibel E (1971) Extracellular lining of bronchioles after perfusion-fixation of rat lungs for electron microscopy. Anat Rec 169:185–200

14. Ebert RV, Terracio MJ (1975) Observation of the secretion of the surface of the bronchioles with scanning electron microscope. Am Rev Respir Dis 112:491–496

15. Breeze R, Turk M (1984) Cellular structure, function and organization in the lower respiratory tract. Environ Health Perspect 55:3–24

16. Hiroshima K, Kohno T, Owada H, Hayashi Y (1987) A morphological study of the effects of ozone on rat lung. I. Short-term exposure. Exp Mol Pathol 47:327–345

17. Plopper CG, Hyde DM, Weir AJ (1983) Centro-acinar alterations in lungs of cats chronically exposed to diesel exhaust. Lab Invest 49:391–399

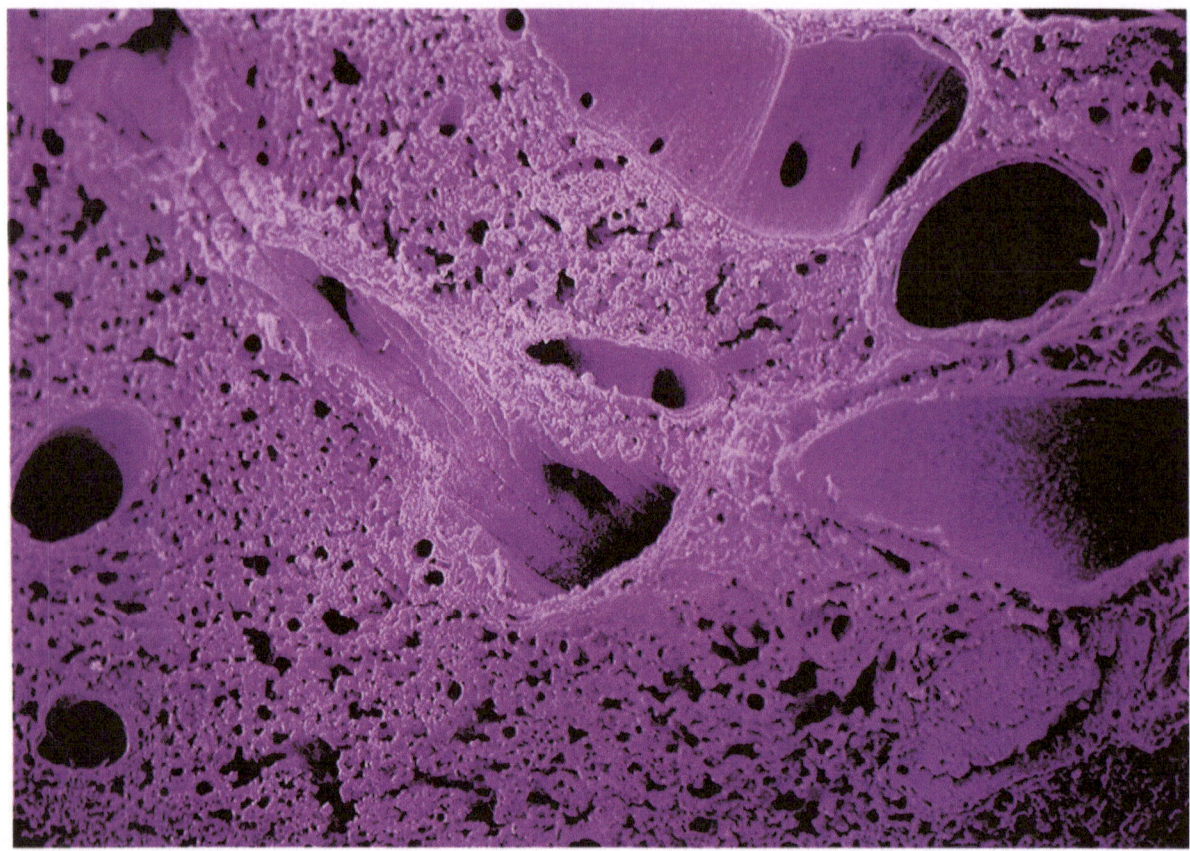

Fig. 5.1. This micrograph shows a section of pulmonary parenchyma at very low magnification. A peripheral bronchiole, the alveolar sacs, and many blood vessels can be seen (×50)

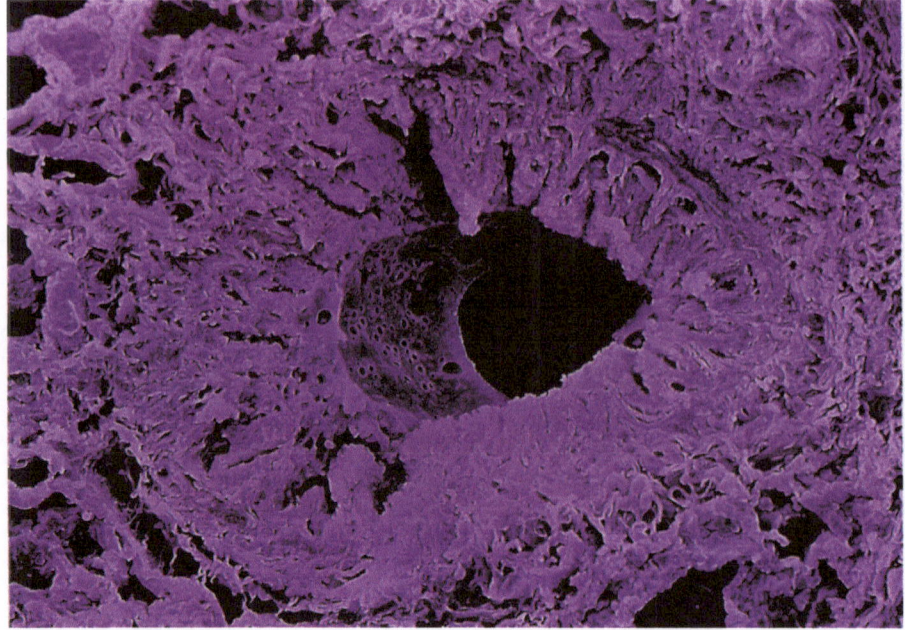

Fig. 5.2. The fundamental structure of the bronchioles can be seen in this micrograph: the columnar epithelium and the underlying basal membrane are easily visible. The oblique section displays the internal surface almost smooth because the layer of the secretion is preserved (×203)

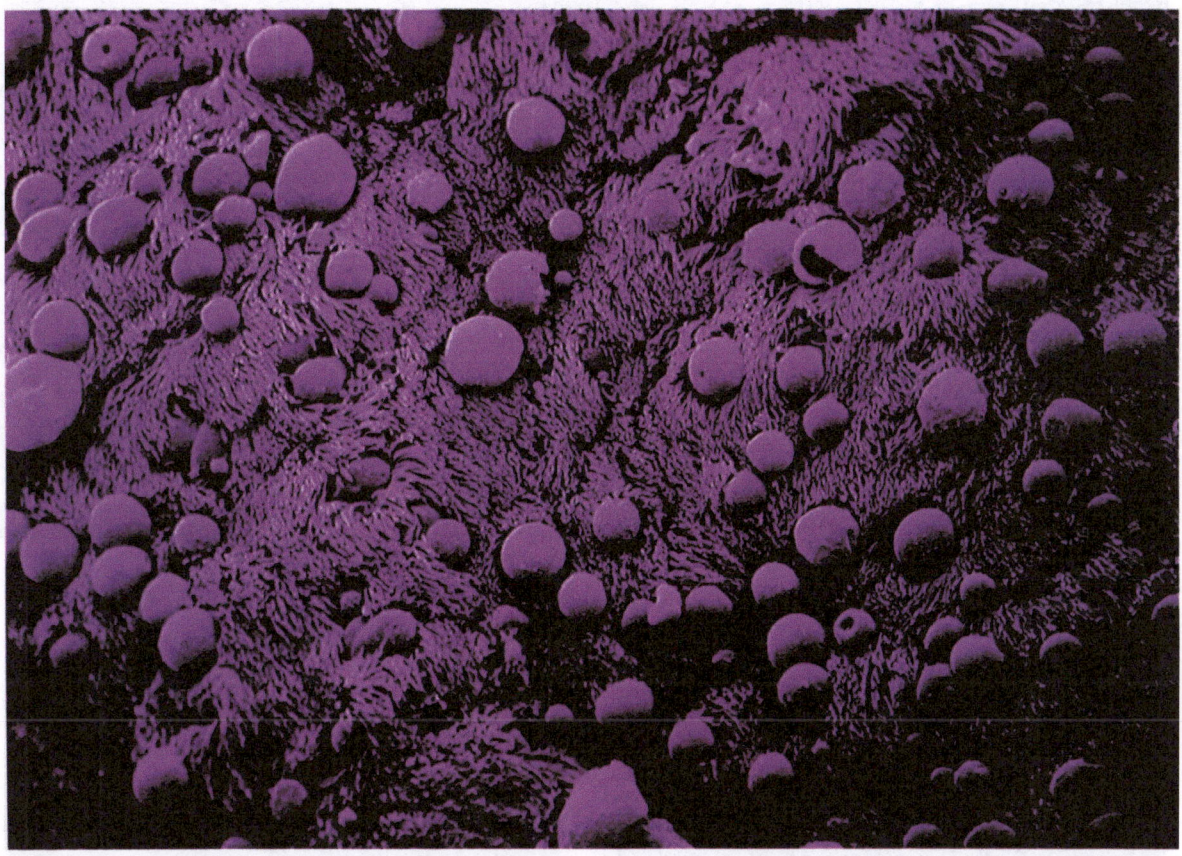

Fig. 5.3. Section of a large bronchiole: numerous ciliated cells and the dome-shaped Clara cells can be observed (×965)

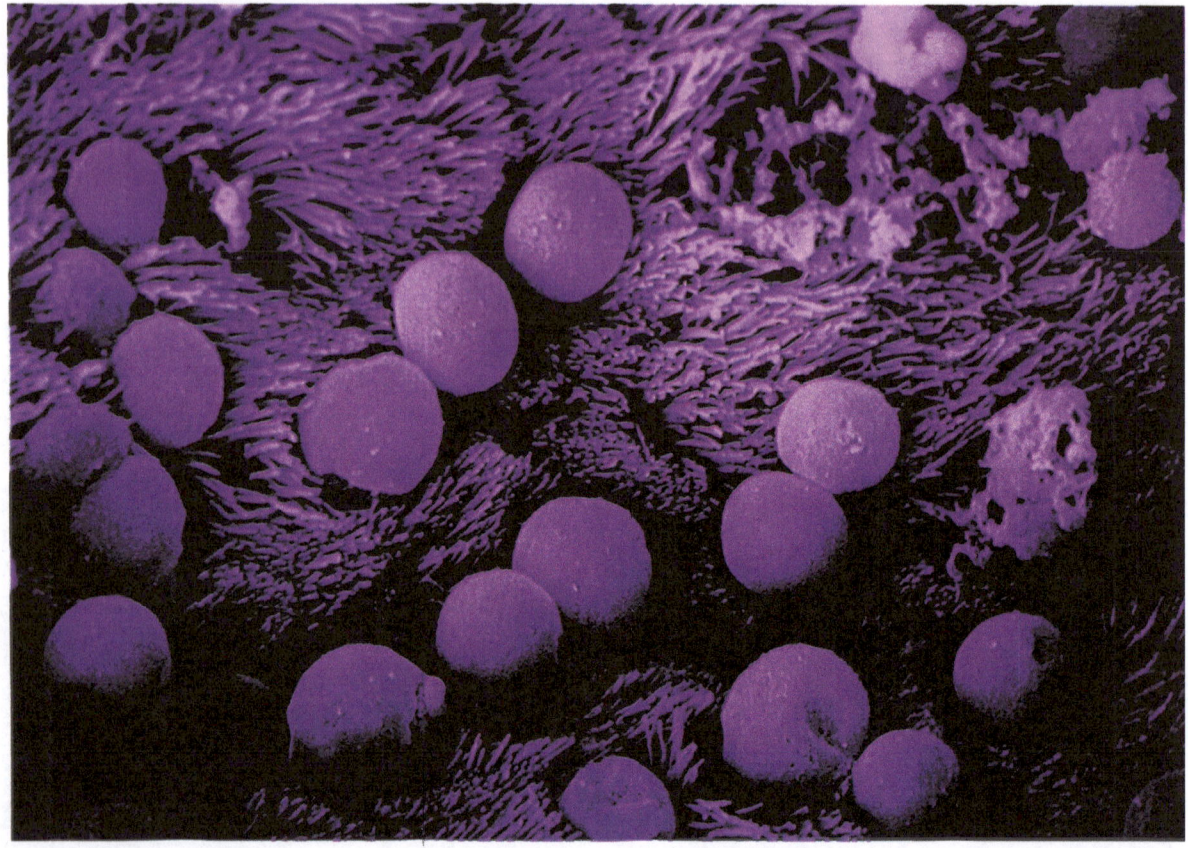

Fig. 5.4. At this magnification, the dissolution of many apices of Clara cells can be seen (×2500)

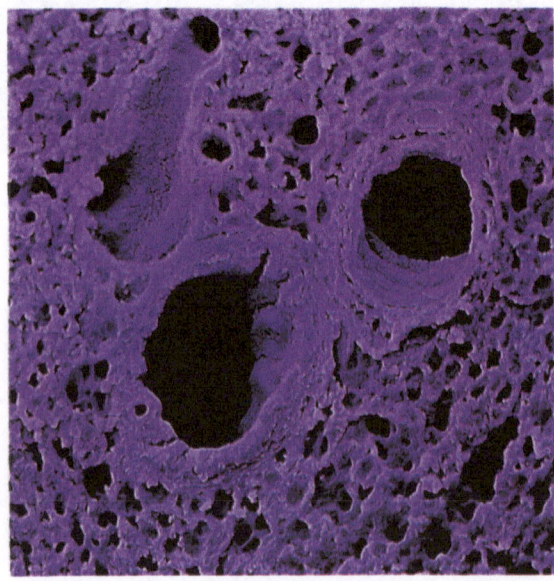

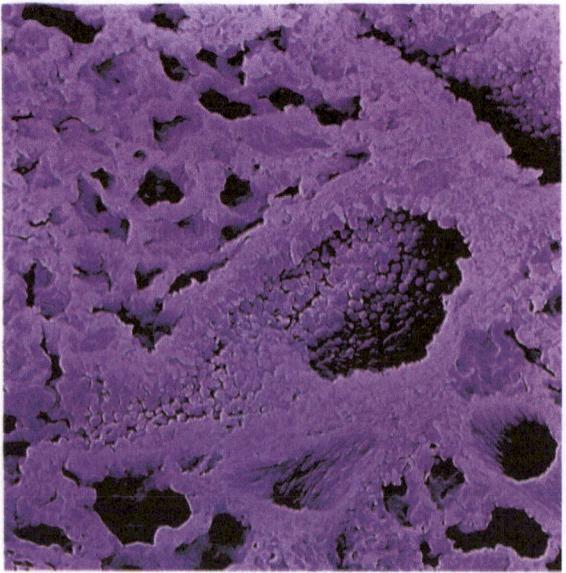

Fig. 5.5. Two peripheral bronchioles and one blood vessel are visible in the pulmonary parenchyma. The bronchiolar epithelium is lined by ciliated and Clara cells and its luminal surface is often roughened and patterned with ridges (×81)

Fig. 5.6. View of peripheral bronchiole sectioned longitudinally and transversally that is mostly lined by Clara cells whose apices markedly bulge into the lumen (×194)

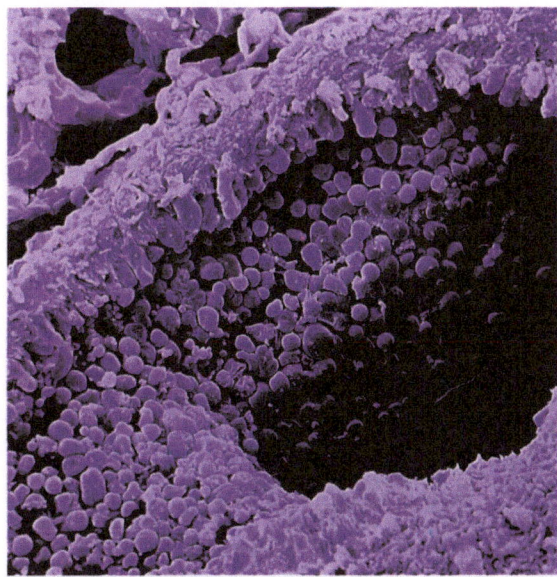

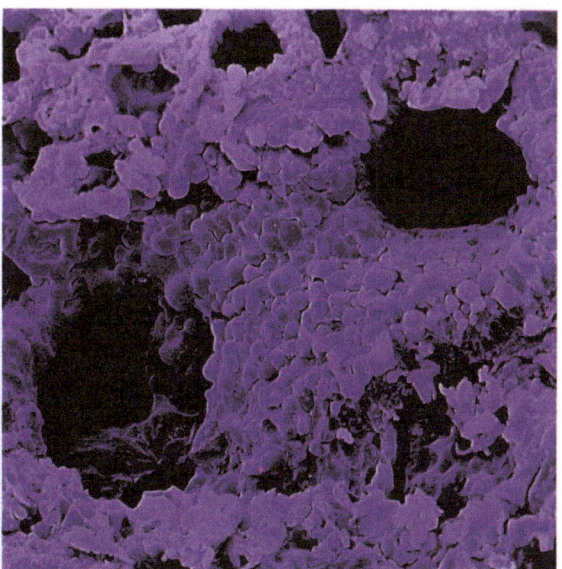

Fig. 5.7. Enlargement of Fig. 5.6. The Clara cells can be seen in frontal and lateral views: they confer a "pebbly" appearance to the bronchiolar luminal surface (×462)

Fig. 5.8. This micrograph depicts the transitional zone between the terminal bronchiole and an alveolar duct. At such a peripheral level, the ciliated cells have nearly disappeared and the epithelium shows the swollen Clara cells, whose granules contain a lipoprotein which is thought to contribute to a surface-active lining layer in the bronchioles (×442)

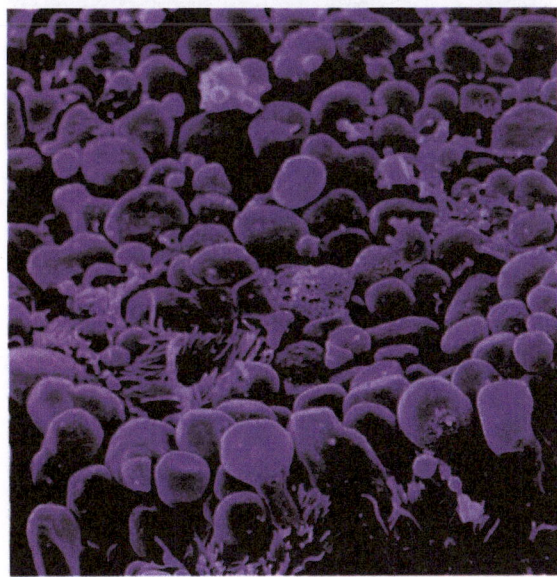

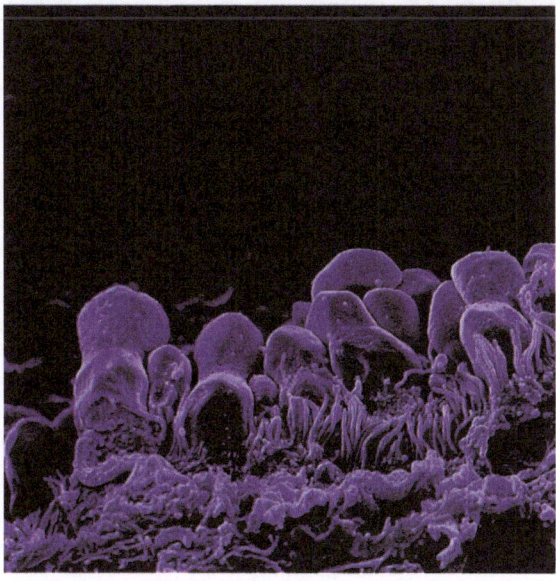

Fig. 5.9. Secretory domes of Clara cells: their dissolution contributes to forming the bronchiolar secretory layer (×1360)

Fig. 5.10. A freeze-fracture of the bronchiolar wall showing the marked protrusion of the apices of Clara cells and the cilia. (×1770)

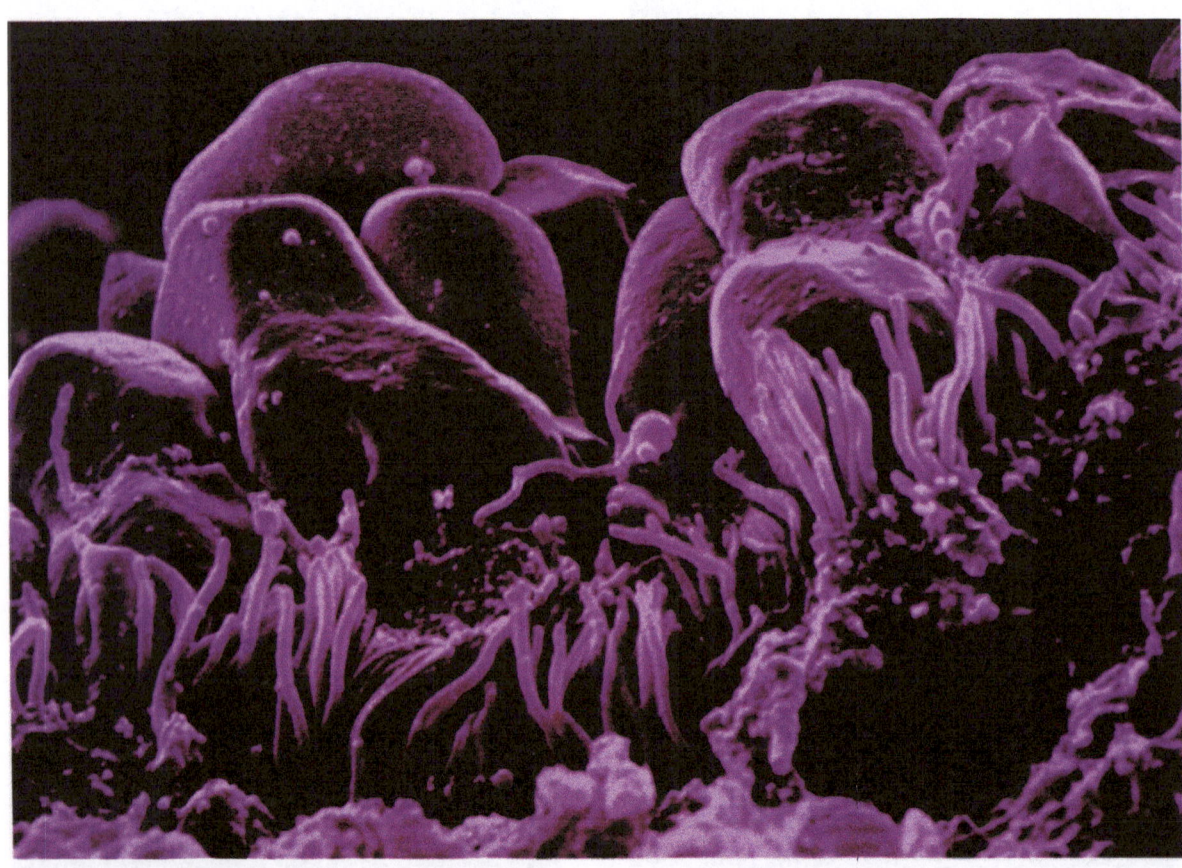

Fig. 5.11. An enlargement of Fig. 5.10 showing the Clara cells in greater detail (×4580)

Chapter 6
Architecture of Alveolar Ducts, Sacs, Alveoli, and Nonresident Cells

L. Allegra and G. Piatti*

Istituto di Malattie Respiratoria, Facoltà di Medicina e Chirurgia,
Università degli Studi di Milano

*Centro di Farmacologia Respiratoria, Facoltà di Medicina e Chirurgia,
Università degli Studi di Milano

Each terminal bronchiole divides into two respiratory bronchioles which have a few alveoli along their course and give rise to several alveolar ducts with walls made entirely of alveoli. The alveolar ducts are followed by the alveolar sacs, which are the sites where many alveoli clusters come together. The alveolus is a terminal anatomical structure of polyhedral conformation in which gas exchange occurs [1]. The dense packing of alveoli (approximately 300 million each, with a diameter of 250 μm) gives the lungs their spongy appearance.

SEM pictures of lung parenchyma at low magnification show a honeycombed structure, and when the angle of the surface cut is appropriate, it beautifully reveals branches of some terminal bronchioles, respiratory bronchioles, and alveolar ducts. The alveoli are separated from each other by extremely thin partitions, the interalveolar septa, in which there is a flexible anastomosis of capillary nets. Sometimes the cut surface reveals the inside of the capillary, and occasionally some erythrocytes can be observed [2].

The alveolar epithelium and its basal membrane are tightly joined to the basal membrane of the endothelium, this structure forming the so-called "alveolus-capillary barrier" (0.2–0.7 μm in thickness). To accomplish its function, the epithelium that covers the alveoli is very flat; the luminal alveolar surface is relatively smooth and lined by a simple squamous epithelium that is a mosaic of two different cell types. Most of the cells (97%) are large alveolar type I cells (50–100 μm) or membranous pneumocytes, which possess a characteristic smooth surface except for a small prominence due to the nucleus [3]. The cytoplasm is so thin that the outlines of erythrocytes in underlying capillaries can be detected in surface views of these cells [4].

Between these squamous cells there are small cuboidal cells with cytoplasmic extensions: these protrude into the lumen, and their lateral borders are often covered by cytoplasmic processes of type I cells. These cells are called alveolar type II cells, or granular pneumocytes, and can be distinguished from adjacent cells by the presence of short microvilli, mostly arranged around the periphery like a "crown" [5]. This cell type is the alveolar secretory cell, which is involved in the sythesis and release of surfactant, a complex of phospholipids rich in lecithin and of proteins that spreads in a thin film on the alveolar surface. While the type I pneumocyte is a highly differentiated cell, and therefore very susceptible to damage by inhaled agents, the type II pneumocyte is multipotential, a stem cell able to proliferate and differentiate into type I pneumocytes, as can be observed in the response to certain forms of alveolar injury. This process requires about 2–6 days, the type II cells form squamous extensions and lose their potential capacity for surfactant synthesis. Type I pneumocytes are joined to each other and to type II pneumocytes by tight junctions and, perhaps, by small gap junctions [6]. The junctions between the cells from the alveolar wall are visible as narrow linear ridges [7].

Another cell type in the alveolar region, one that is only rarely found, is the brush cell, also called the type III pneumocyte: it does not differ mophologically from those in other airways, but its function is unknown.

Within the three-dimensional alveolar structure, SEM also reveals small circular or oral openings (10–15 μm in diameter) which cross the interalveolar septum and permit communication between adjacent alveoli, preventing their collapses when there is a bronchiolar obstruction and equalizing air pressure within the lung. These are called the pores of Kohn [8]. Their variability in shape and size may result from the phase of breathing, although such changes are poorly documented [9]. There are also bronchiolar-alveolar communications called Lambert's pores (canals) that permit a further collateral ventilation of the alveoli.

The alveolar spaces also contain free (or non-resident) cells with phagocytic activity, the alveolar macrophages. These are conspicuous cell population lining the alveolar surface [10, 11] and are transiently attached to the surface of the alveolar epithelium by pseudopodia. It seems that they can crawl over this surface by ameboid movement. They are derived from blood monocytes via interstitial macrophages, and from the interstitial tissue they migrate into the alveoli. These cells are very useful for removal of inhaled foreign particles, such debris or microorganisms, from the lung. Particulate material is in fact digested by their intracellular lysosomes. Some macrophages penetrate into the interstitium and can be visualized here as deposits of pigment; others are cleared with the airway mucus. Alveolar phagocytes are also involved in removal of surfactant. The surface morphology and shapes of macrophage cells are heterogeneous: resting macrophages are oval, with irregular cytoplasmic processes that become more elongated and folded when the cell is motile and phagocytic [12]. Many macrophages can sometimes be seen lodged within the pores of Kohn, migrating between adjacent alveoli. A bronchoalveolar lavage contains numerous free alveolar macrophages (about 70% of total cells recovered): flat cells, which are active phagocytes, and round cells, which are relatively quiescent, can be discerned in approximately equal numbers [13].

The alveolar epithelium is also coated by a thin extracellular layer that is only poorly preserved with the usual fixation techniques for electron microscopy. Only vascular perfusion can demonstrate this lining, called the surfactant. The alveolar surfactant forms a continuous sheet from alveoli to terminal bronchioles and is a mixture of phospholipids and proteins. The phospholipids are synthesized by type II pneumocytes and released by neurocrine secretion. The source of the proteins may be the Clara cells, but this has not yet been conclusively established. The surfactant is a mixture of surface-active substances that prevents alveolar collapse by lowering the surface tension. Pulmonary surfactant is turned over rather rapidly: part of it leaves the already occupied spaces over the terminal bronchioles, part is engulfed by alveolar macrophages, and another part, inactivated surfactant, may be recycled through the type II pneumocytes. In addition to stabilizing the alveoli, surfactant physically protects the alveolar epithelium from viruses and bacteria, reducing their adhesiveness [14].

Pulmonary parenchyma is an excellent subject for investigation by SEM because of the spectacular three-dimensional structure of alveoli, but a suitable fixation technique must be used to demonstrate the above-mentioned constituents.

References

1. Staub NC, Albertine KH (1988) The structure of the lungs relative to their principal function. In: Murray H, Nadel J (eds) Textbook of respiratory medicine. Saunders, London, pp 12–46
2. Maisin JR, Van Gorp U, De Saint-Georges L (1982) The ultrastructure of the lung after exposure to ionizing radiation as seen be transmission and scanning electron microscopy. Scanning Electron Microsc 1:403–412
3. Williams MC (1990) The alveolar epithelium. Structure and study by immunocytochemistry. In: Schraufnagel DE (ed) Electron microscopy of the lung, vol 48. Dekker, New York, pp 121–147
4. Greenwood MF, Holland P (1972) The mammalian respiratory tract surface. A scanning electron microscopic study. Lab Invest 27:296–304
5. Fishman AP (1988) Pulmonary diseases and disorders, vol 1, McGraw-Hill, New York, pp 11–44
6. Bartles H, Oestern HJ, Voss-Wermbter G (1980) Communicating-occluding junction complexes in the alveolar epithelium. Am Rev Respir Dis 121:1017–1024
7. Kessel RG, Kardon RH (1979) Tissue and organs: a text-atlas of SEM. Freeman, San Francisco, pp 203–217
8. Davis ML, Lewandowski J, Dodson RF (1984) Morphology and ultrastructure of the distal airway epithelium in the guinea pig. Anat Rec 209:509–522

9. Groniowsky J, Walski M, Biczysko W (1972) Application of scanning electron microscopy for study of the lung parenchyma. J Ultrastruct Res 37:473–481

10. Breeze R, Turk M (1984) Cellular structure, function and organization in the lower respiratory tract. Environ Health Perspect 55:3–24

11. Green GM, Jakab GJ, Low RB, Davis GS (1977) Defense mechanisms of the respiratory membrane. Am Rev Respir Dis 115:479–549

12. Andrews PM (1979) The respiratory system. In: Hodges GM, Hallowes RC (eds) Biomedical applications of SEM, vol 1. Academic, London, pp 177–202

13. Davis GS (1979) Functional and physiologic correlates of human alveolar macrophage cell shape and surface morphology. Chest 75 (Suppl):280–282

14. Morgenroth K (1979) Il surfattante polmonare. De Gruyter, Berlin

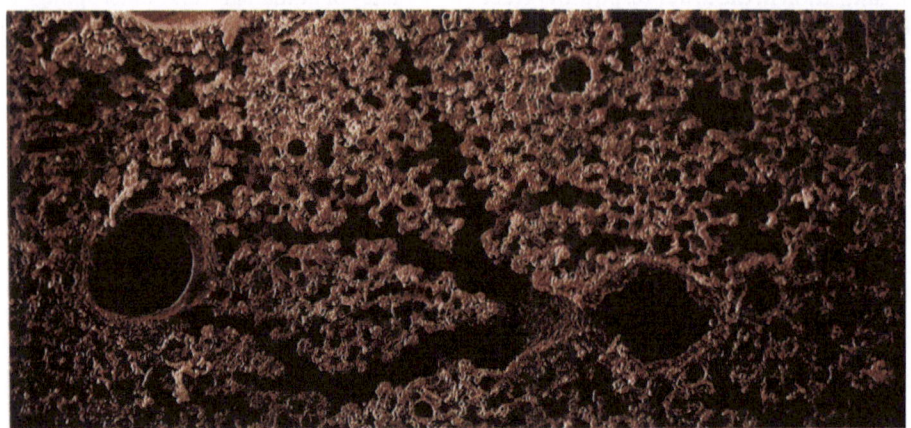

Fig. 6.1. Pulmonary tissue, at low magnification, showing many blood vessels and a peripheral bronchiole branching into several alveolar ducts (×81)

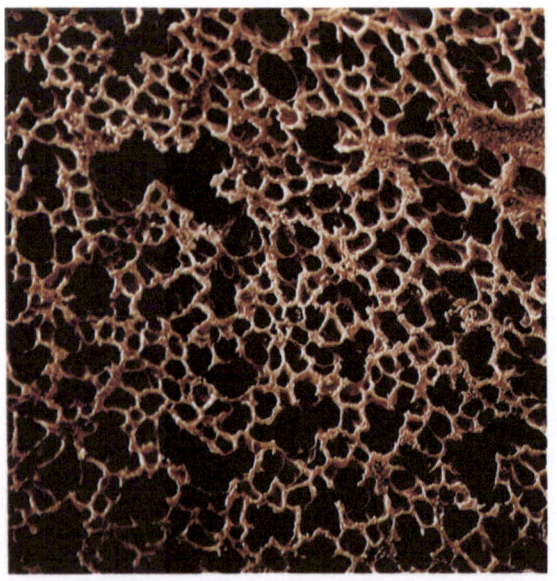

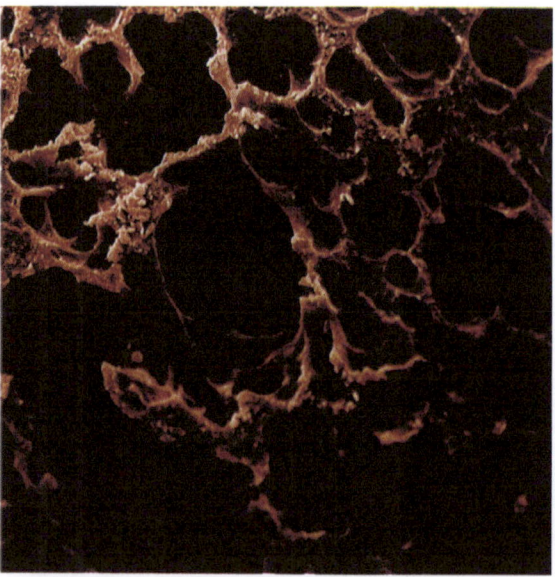

Fig. 6.2. Appearance of pulmonary parenchyma. The spongy aspect is due to the presence of many alveolar ducts (×71)

Fig. 6.3. Detail of part of the Fig. 6.2 at higher magnification (×200)

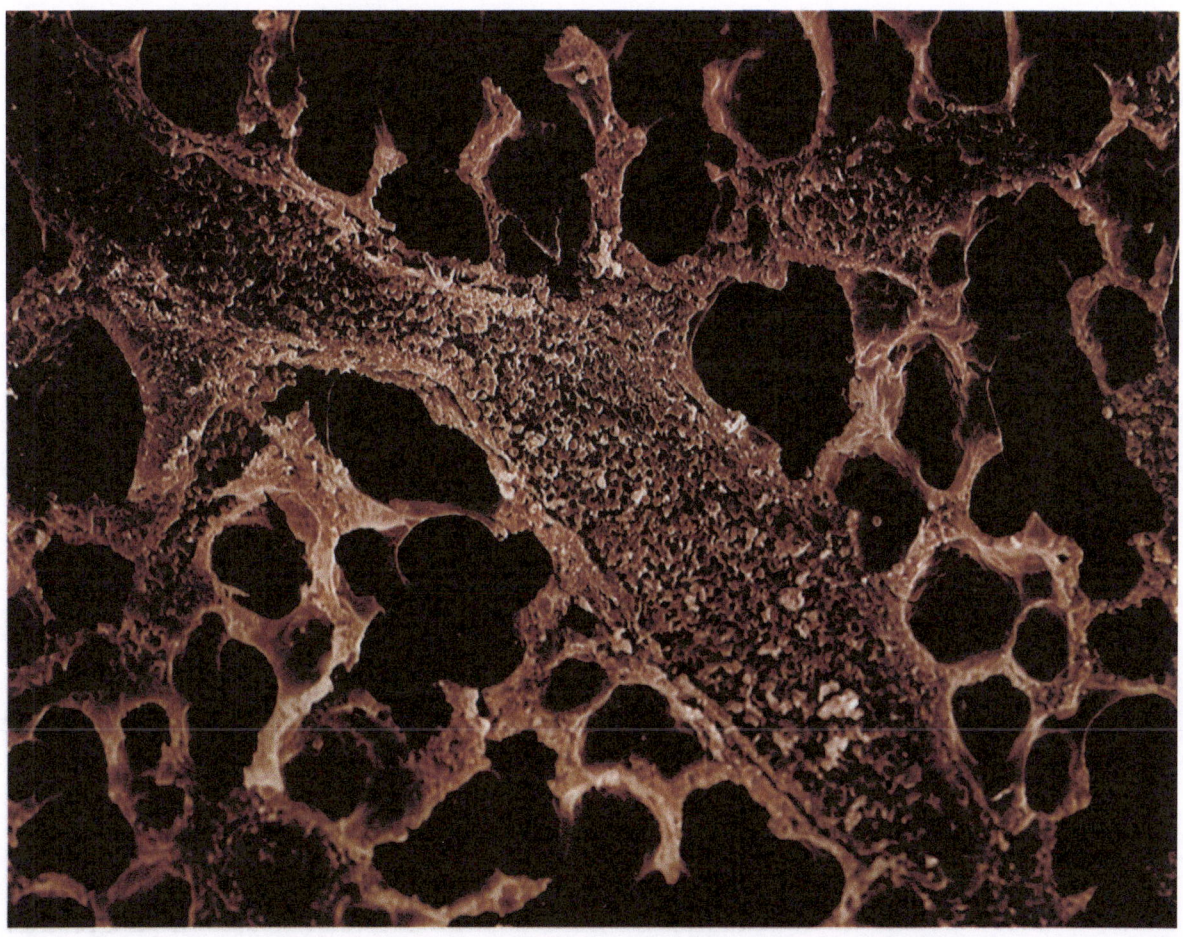

Fig. 6.4. Scanning electron micrograph of a blood vessel in the pulmonary parenchyma filled with densely packed erythrocytes ($\times$194)

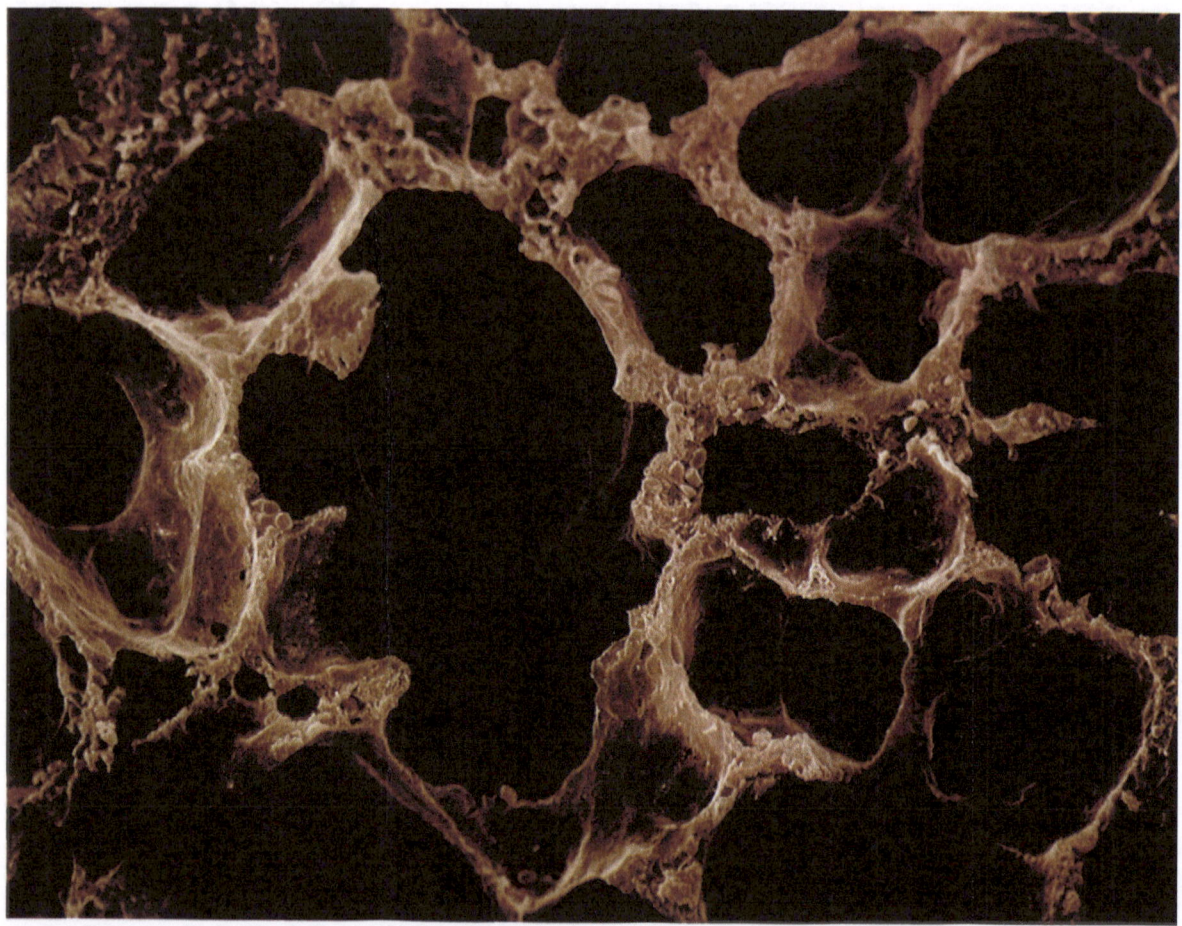

Fig. 6.5. This section shows a close-up of an alveolar duct which opens into many alveoli (×372)

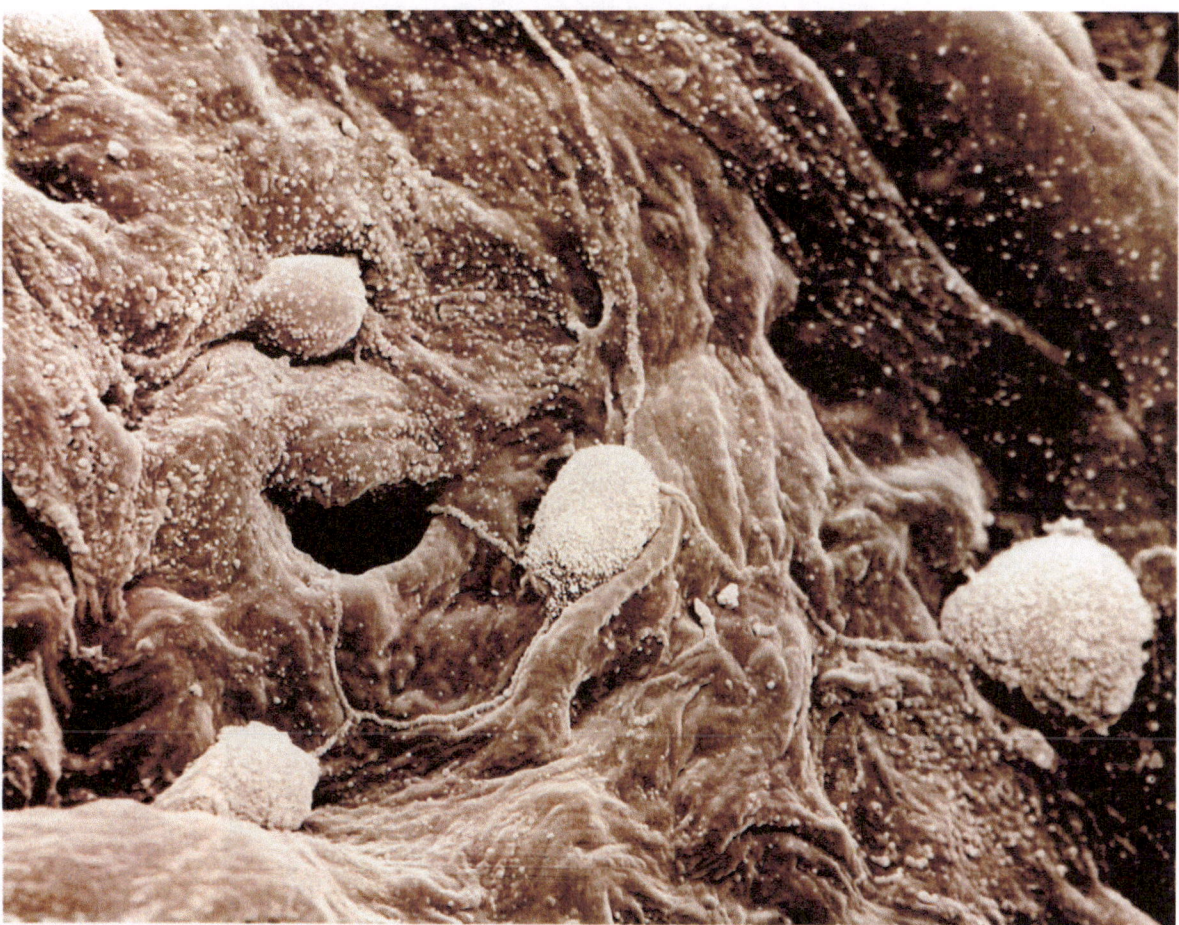

Fig. 6.6. The alveolar surface is a "mosaic" of two different cell types: the large and flat type I pneumocytes and the type II pneumocytes, which are joined to each other by junctional complexes visible on the surface as linear ridges. A pore of Kohn is visible as a black hole in the *central area* of the micrograph (×1770)

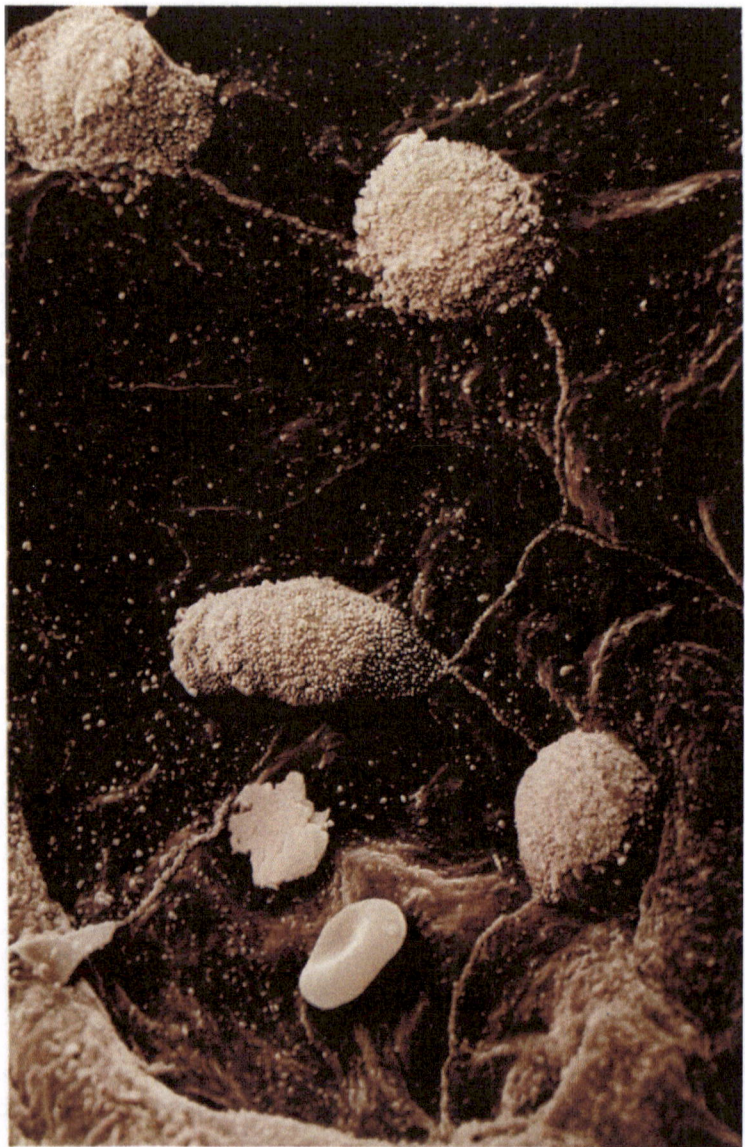

Fig. 6.7. The type II pneumocytes protrude into the alveolar cavity and their surfaces are covered by small microvilli. The tight junctions between the cells are clearly visible ($\times$2020)

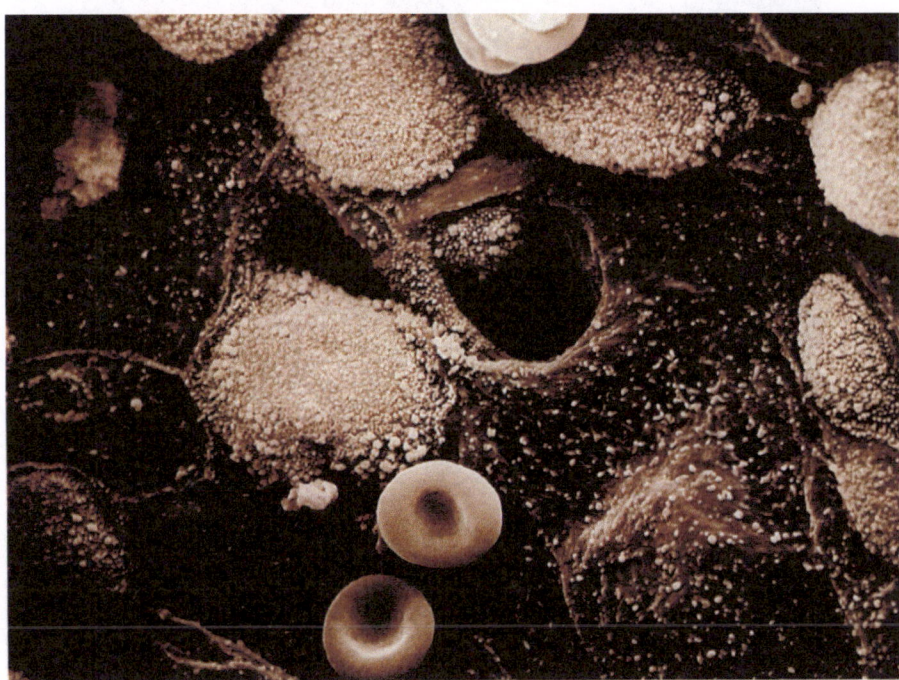

Fig. 6.8. Internal view of an alveolus which allows a comparison between the dimensions of the type II pneumocytes and the two erythrocytes located in the *lower part* of the micrograph (×2620)

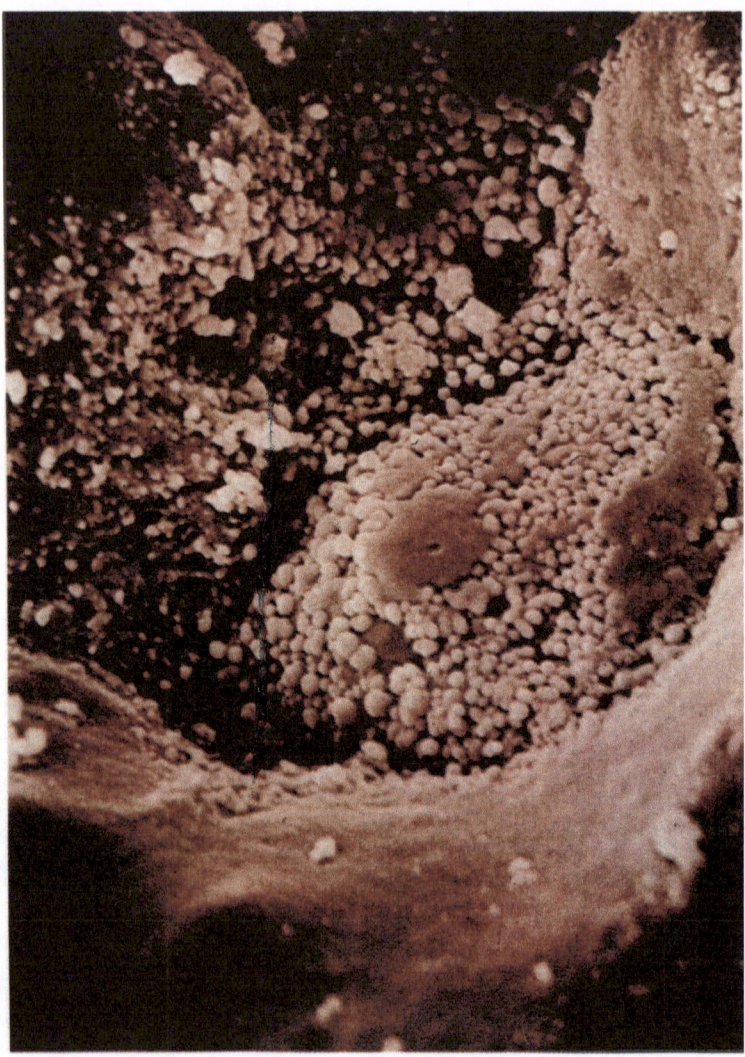

Fig. 6.9. High magnification of a type II pneumocyte in secretory
phase while it is releasing its products (×9600)

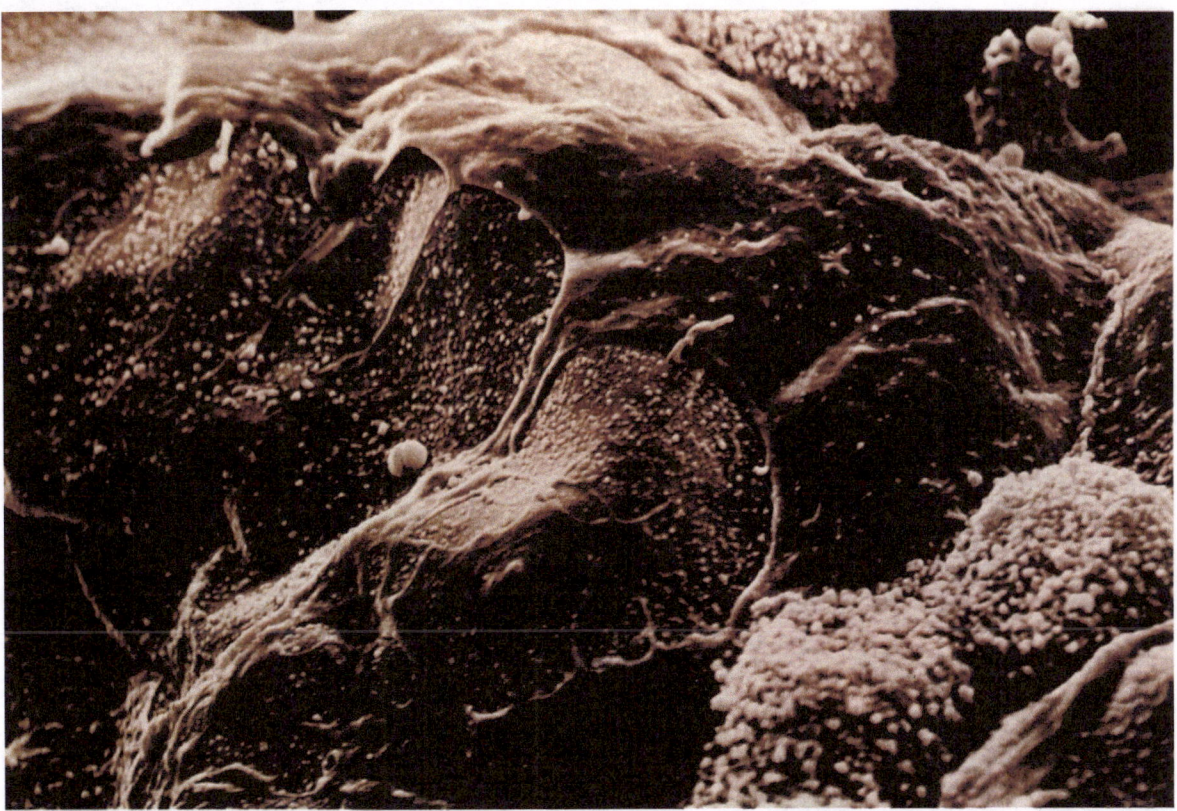

Fig. 6.10. The alveolar surface seen partially covered by the surfactant layer ($\times$3240)

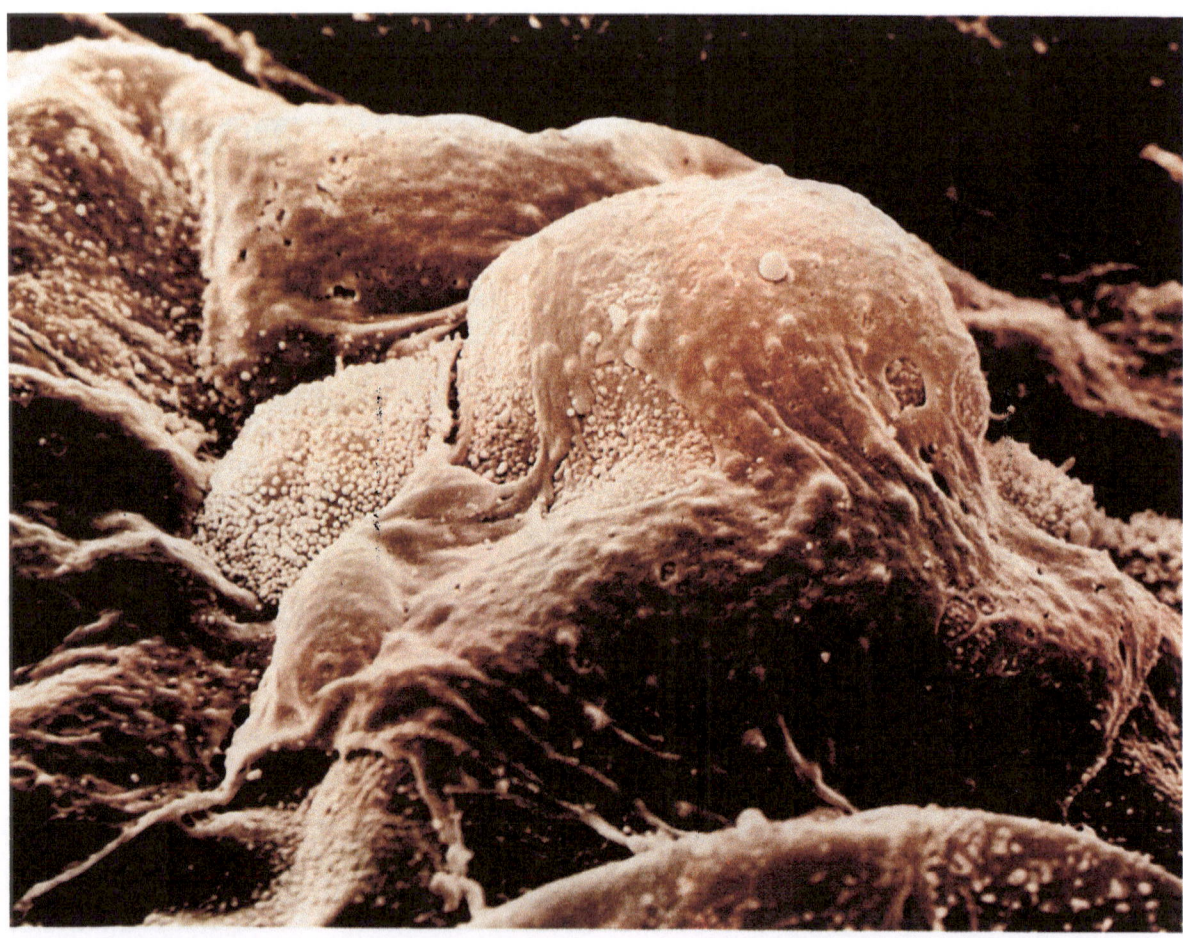

Fig. 6.11. *Central* is a close-up view of a dome-shaped type II pneumocyte
covered by a thin layer of surfactant (×2720)

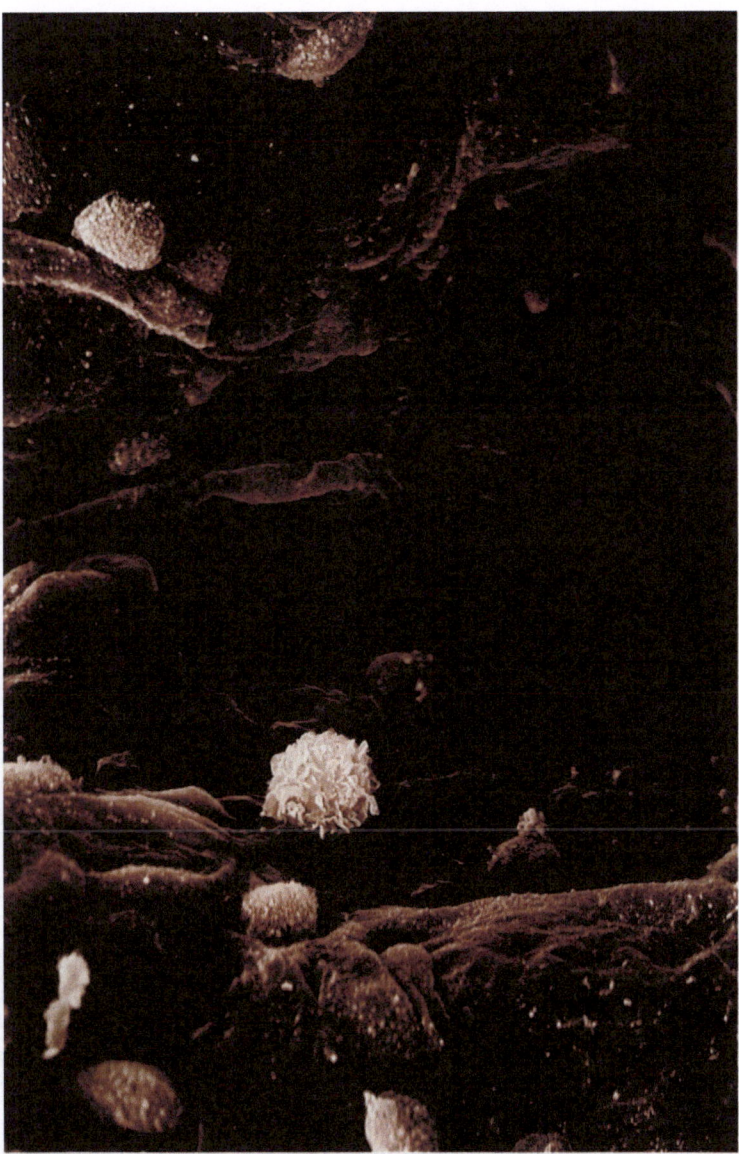

Fig. 6.12. Internal view of an alveolar cavity with an alveolar macrophage lying on the alveolar surface (×1050)

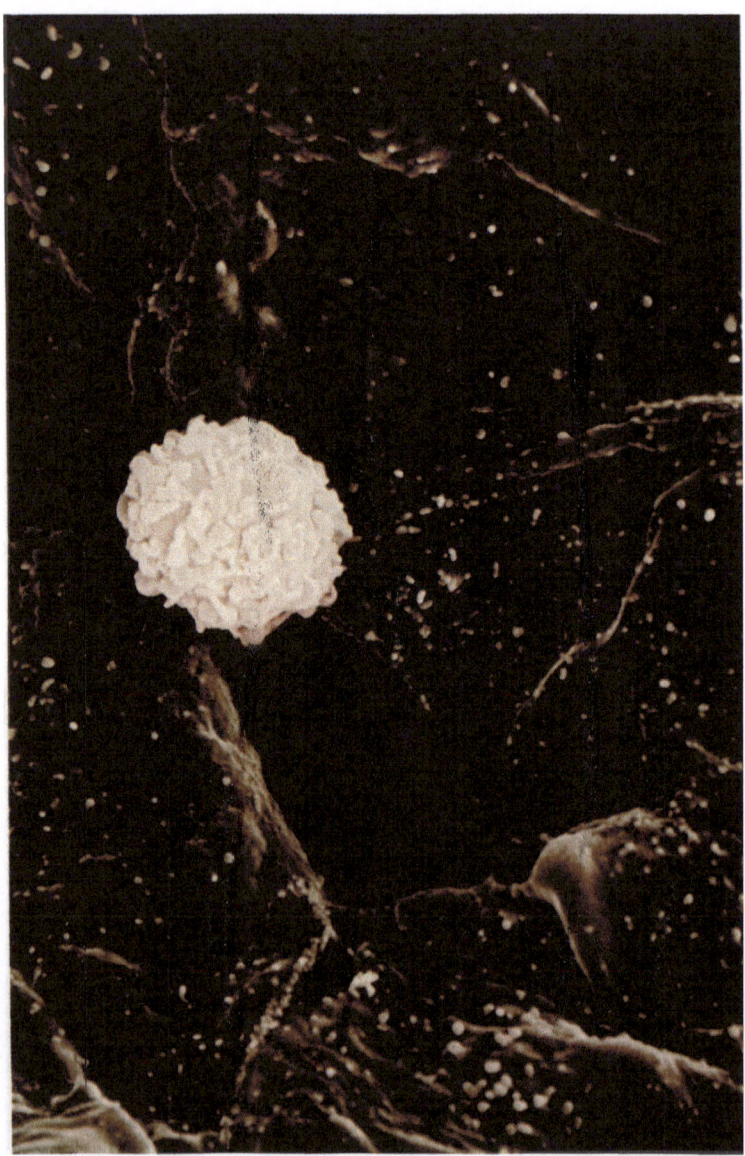

Fig. 6.13. The round clear cell is an alveolar macrophage on the edge of a pore of Kohn (black hole), probably as it is passing through into another alveolus (×4020)

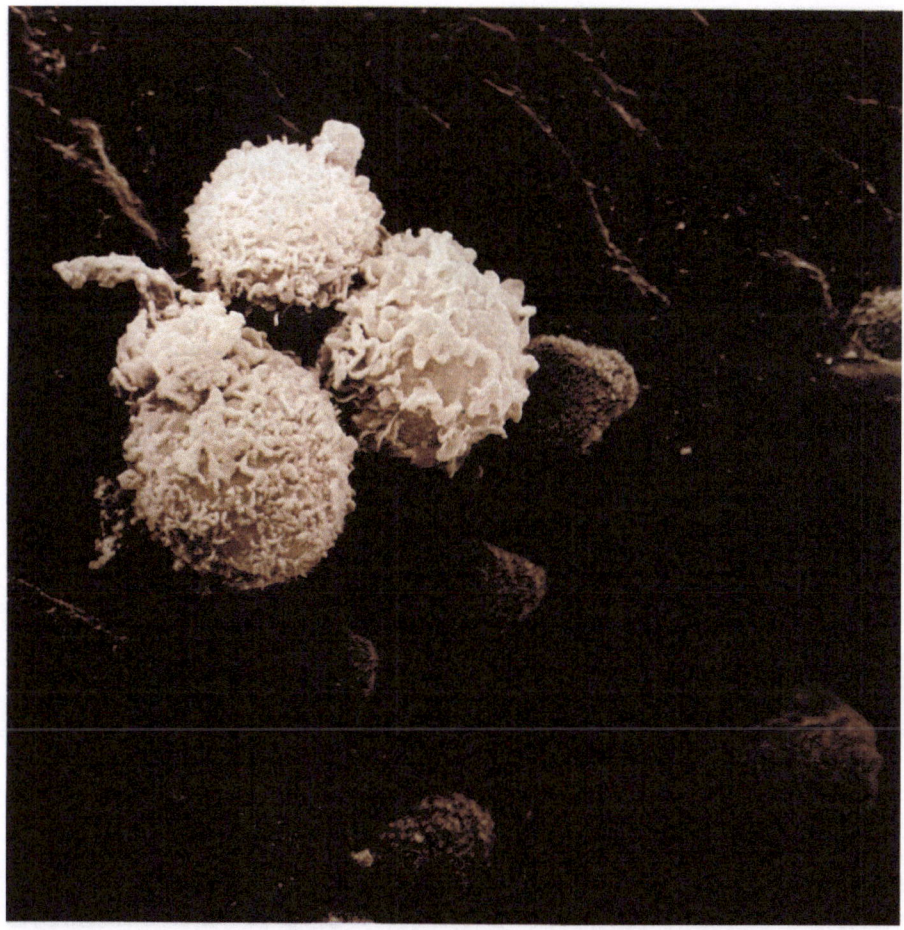

Fig. 6.14. A group of alveolar macrophages displaying various degrees of microfolding on their surfaces ($\times$1550)

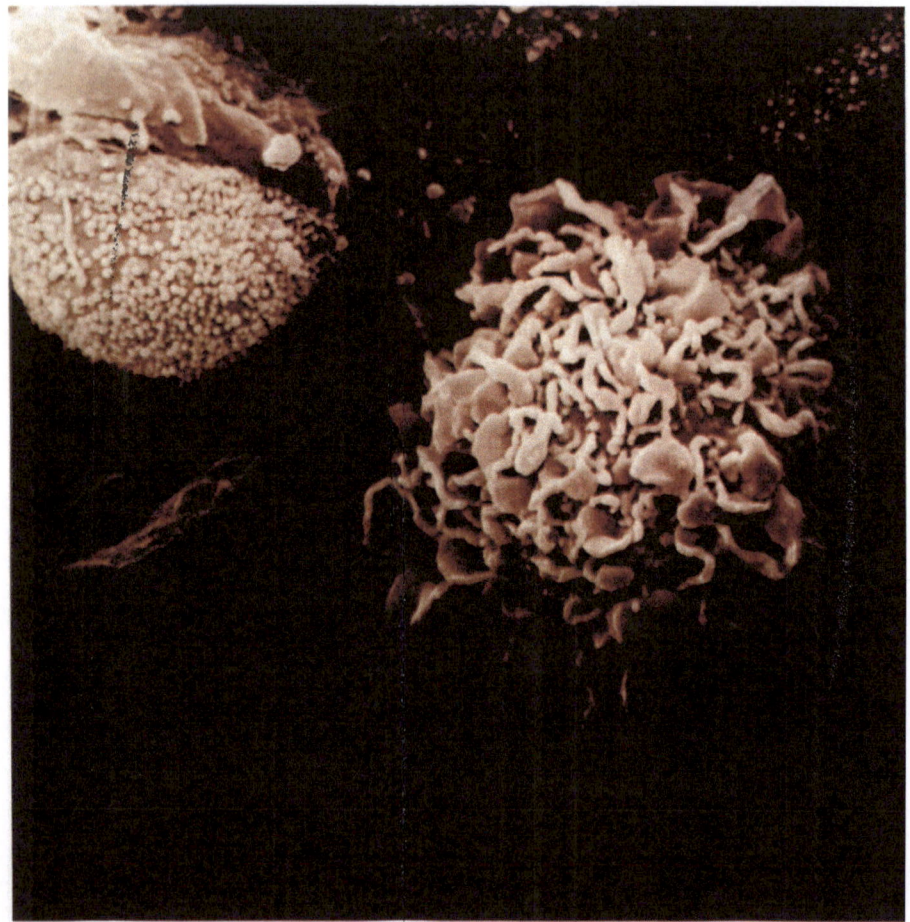

Fig. 6.15. Close-up of a macrophage showing many microfolds protruding
from its surface (×4020)

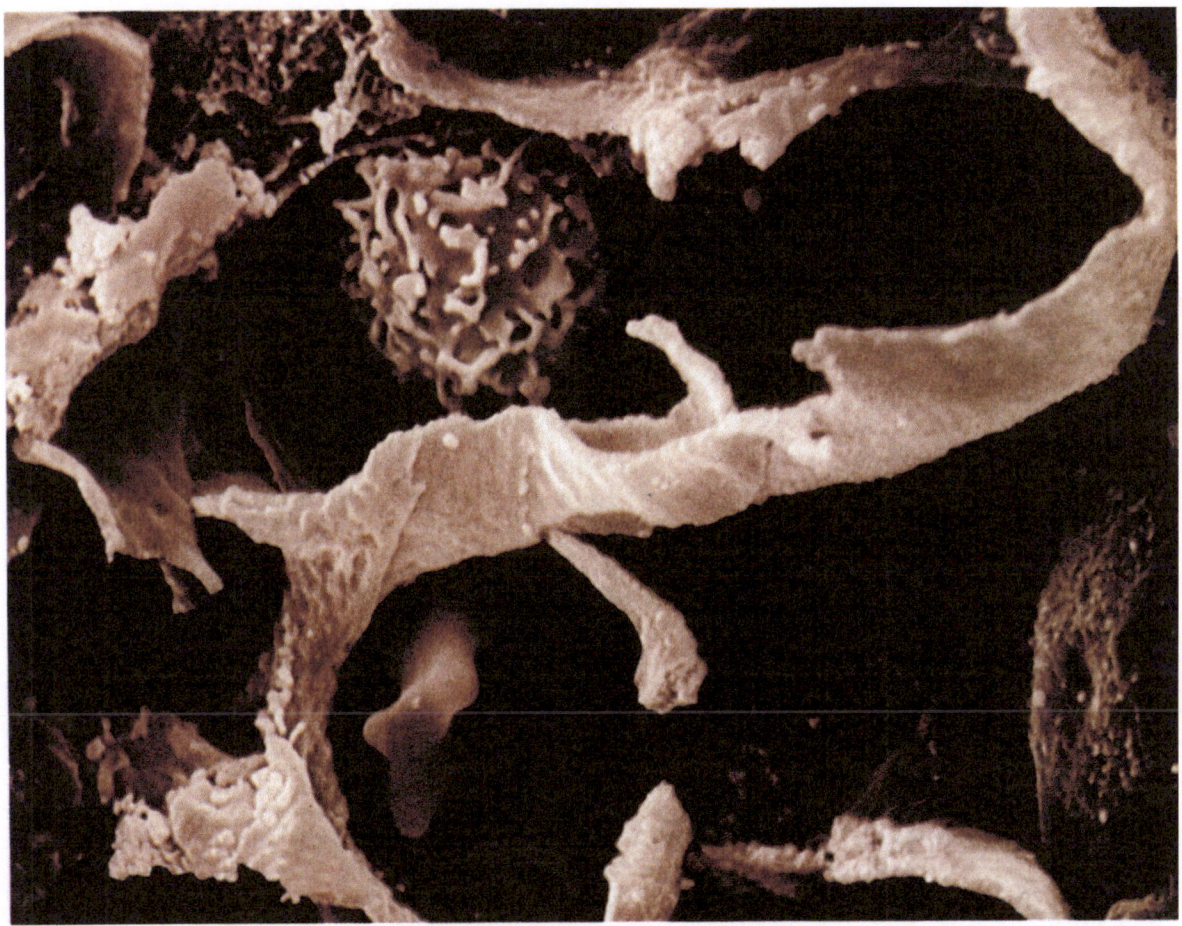

Fig. 6.16. This picture shows an alveolar septum with a trapped white blood cell *(above)* and a red blood cell *(below)* ($\times$5000)

Chapter 7
Damage to Airway Epithelium

P. C. Braga, L. Allegra*, and G. Piatti

Centro di Farmacologia Respiratoria, Facoltà di Medicina e Chirurgia,
Università degli Studi di Milano

* Istituto di Malattie Respiratoria, Facoltà di Medicina e Chirurgia,
Università degli Studi di Milano

Ciliated cells and goblet cells are the cells most exposed to external noxae, and thus more subject to damage. In chronic bronchitic disease and in other pulmonary diseases in which there is abnormal mucus production, the goblet cells appear swollen and increased in number, while cilia are often nonuniformly glued to each other by mucus. During bacterial and viral infections marked changes have been observed in the "ciliated carpet". Initially there is a partial sloughing of isolated ciliated cells and, mainly during viral infection, also loss of cilia, more severe in the bronchioli and small intrapulmonary bronchi than in the major bronchi. This loss of cilia destroys the ciliary carpet on the luminal surface of these airways and exposes the microvilli [1]. The exact mechanism of ciliary loss has not been determined. The damage is not uniform, as intact areas are still visible scattered throughout the respiratory mucosae, near damaged areas.

After a variable period of time (72–96 h), increased sloughing of epithelial cells and loss of cilia result in mucosal damage, and provide suitable conditions for infecting microorganisms to invade the respiratory mucosa extensively (there is no effective mucociliary clearance) and cross the mucosal barrier of the respiratory tract [2–5]. At this time, larger areas of denuded mucosa can be seen, resulting in a great increase in the ability of bacteria to colonize through their adhesiveness, as this is no longer prevented by an effective mucociliary clearance mechanism.

The appearance of macrophages on the surface of damaged bronchiolar and alveolar epithelium [1] is early evidence of repair. Macrophages, epithelial cells, and fibroblasts are all involved in the repair process [1]. Recovery of the epithelia takes many days and is usually complete within 2 weeks or more [6].

Chronic infections with repeated injury of ciliated epithelium can led to ultrastructural defects in the respiratory tract cilia [7, 8]. Ultrastructural dysmorphology of cilia is also seen in other conditions, such as Kartagener's syndrome [9], immotile-cilia syndrome [10, 11], bronchopulmonary dysplasia [12], and other forms of ciliary dyskinesia [13]. These conditions are characterized by ultrastructural defects in the internal ciliary axonemes, which can be observed by TEM but not by SEM because generally the external shape of the cilia does not differ from that seen normally. It has been suggested that the presence of these abnormal cilia may be of pathogenic significance and that they may be responsible for the decreased mucociliary function found in Kartagener's syndrome, bronchiectasis, and chronic bronchitis [14].

Only a few studies have been done on the specific action of different chemical or physical noxae on cilia morphology, but it has been reported that physical agents such as ionizing radiation [15, 16], heat [17], chemicals [18–20], and inhaled gases [21] can all injure and produce changes in cilia morphology.

References

1. Bryson DG, McNulty MS, McCracken RN, Cush PF (1983) Ultrastructural features of experimental parainfluenza type 3 virus pneumonia in calves. J Comp Pathol 93:397–413

2. Moorthy ARS, Spradbrow PB (1985) The effect of mycoplasmas and acholeplasmas of equine origin on organ cultures of chicken-embryo trachea. J Comp Pathol 95:209–216

3. Gabridge MG, Bright MJ, Richards HR (1982) Scanning electron microscopy of mycoplasma pneumoniae on the membrane of individual ciliated tracheal cell. In Vitro 18:55–62

4. Bertrand B, Degen A (1983) Étude de la clearance mucociliare en clinique courante et anomalies ciliaires en microscopie électronique. Acta Oto-Rinho-Otorhinolaryngol Belg 37:662–671

5. Johnson AP, Clark JB, Osborn MF (1983) Scanning electron microscopy of the interaction between Haemophilus influenzae and organ cultures of rat trachea. J Med Microbiol 16:477–482

6. Azoulay-Dupuis E, Lambre CR, Soler P, Moreu J, Thibon M (1984) Lung alterations in guinea-pigs infection with influenza virus. J Comp Pathol 94:273–283

7. Howell JI, Schochet SS, Goldman AS (1980) Ultrastructural defects of respiratory tract cilia associated with chronic infections. Arch Pathol Lab Med 140:52–55

8. Neustein H, Church J, Cohens S (1979) Dysmorphology of cilia associated with chronic suppurative respiratory disease. JAMA 214:2423

9. Theopold HM, Jakneke V, Schinko I (1984) Zur Feinstruktur der Zilien bei Kartagener-Syndrom. Laryngorhinotologie 63:33–40

10. Afzelius BA (1981) "Immotile-cilia" syndrome and ciliary abnormalities induced by infection and injury. Am Rev Respir Dis 124:107–109

11. Schneberger EE, McCormack J, Issenberg HK, Schuster SR, Gerald PS (1980) Heterogeneity of ciliary morphology in the immotile-cilia syndrome in man. J Ultrastruct Res 73:34–43

12. Lee RMKW, Rossman CM, O'Brodvich H, Forrest JB, Newhouse MT (1984) Ciliary defects associated with the development of bronchopulmonary dysplasia. Ciliary motility and ultrastructure. Am Rev Respir Dis 129:190–193

13. Rossman CM, Lee RMKW, Forrest JB, Newhouse MT (1984) Nasal ciliary ultrastructure and function in patients with primary ciliary dyskinesia compared with that in normal subjects and in subjects with various respiratory diseases. Am Rev Respir Dis 129:161–167

14. Fox B, Bull TB, Makey AR, Rawbone R (1981) The significance of ultrastructural abnormalities of human cilia. Chest 80 (Suppl):796–799

15. Albertsson M, Baldetorp B, Hakanssin CH, Meckleburg CV (1984) The effects of 10 Gy single-dose irradiation of the ciliated epithelium measured during a one-to-ten day following irradiation. Scaning Electron Microsc 2:813–824

16. Albertsson M (1985) Dose-response studies of single dose ionizing radiation on the ciliated epithelium of the trachea of the rabbit. Acta Radiol Oncol 24:433–443

17. Meecklenburg CV, Mercke U, Hakansson CH, Toremalm NG (1974) Morphological changes in ciliary cells due to heat exposure. A scanning electron microscopy study. Cell Tissue Res 148:45–46

18. Albertsson N, Hakansson CH (1988) Changes in the tracheal ciliated cells in rabbit treated by cisdiamminedichloroplatinum (II) as studies by electron microscopy. Scanning Microsc 2:2173–2179

19. Dickett KE, Schiller SL, Girard PR, Kennedy JR (1986) The effects of gossypol on the ultrastructure and function of tracheal ciliated cells. J Submicrosc Cytol 18:117–125

20. Schiff LJ, Byrne MM, Elliot SF, More SJ, Ketels KV, Graham JA (1981) Response of hamster trachea in organ culture to mount St. Helens volcano ash. Scanning Electron Microsc 2:164–178

21. Overton JH, Miller FJ (1988) Absorption of inhaled reactive gases. In: Gardner DE, Crapo JD, Massaro EJ (eds) Toxicology of the lung. Raven, New York, pp 477–507

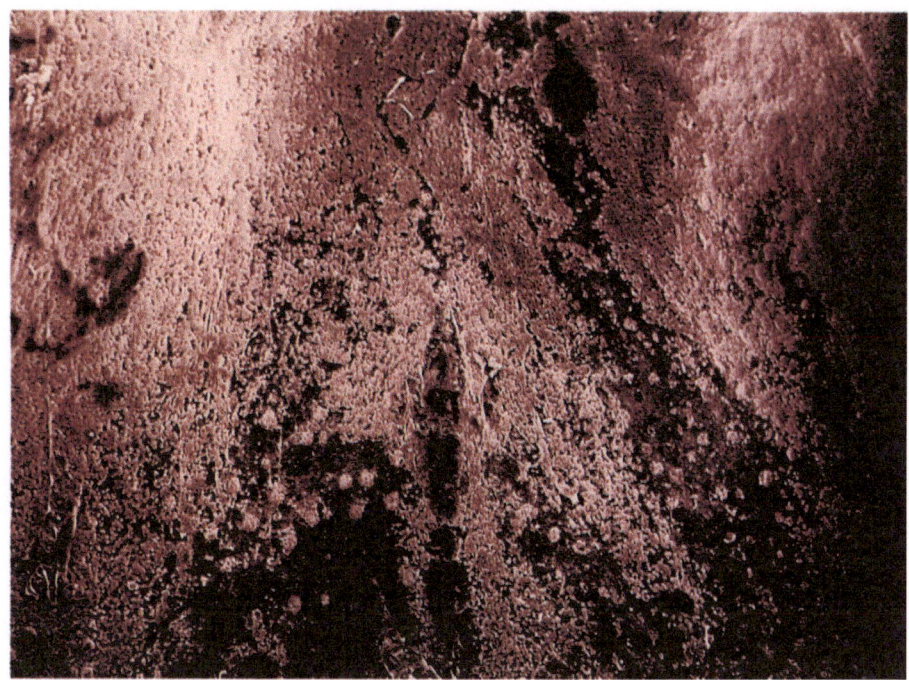

Fig. 7.1. Scanning electron microscopy of the bronchial mucosa from above. At very low magnification a rather extensive damaged area, of respiratory epithelium can be seen (the *dark* zones) (×19)

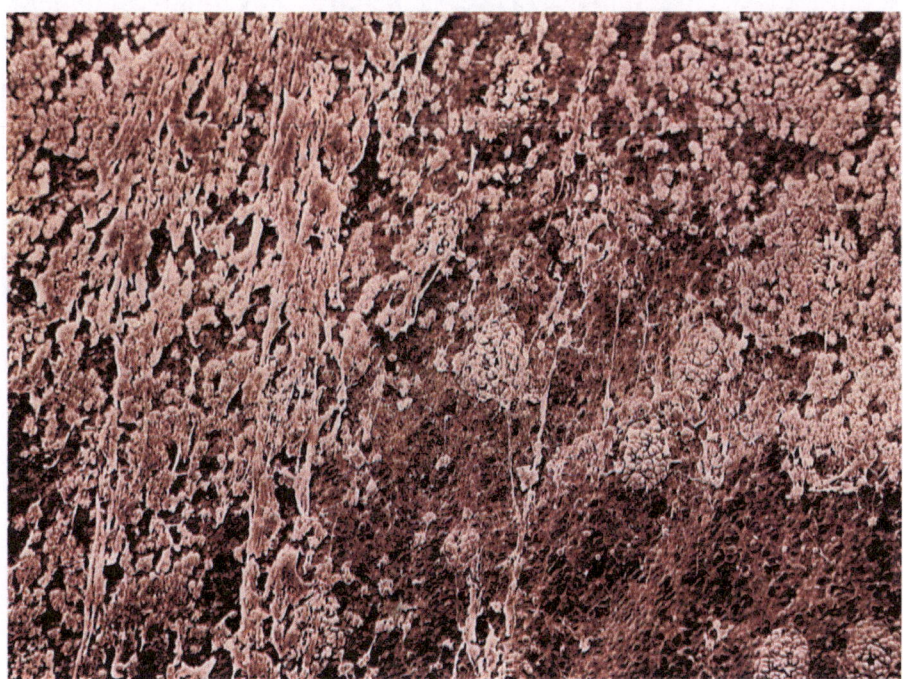

Fig. 7.2. Bronchial mucosa showing the zone of transition between ciliated and damaged nonciliated epithelium where scattered tufts of ciliated cells are still present. On the *left,* a few mucous filaments are visible (×78)

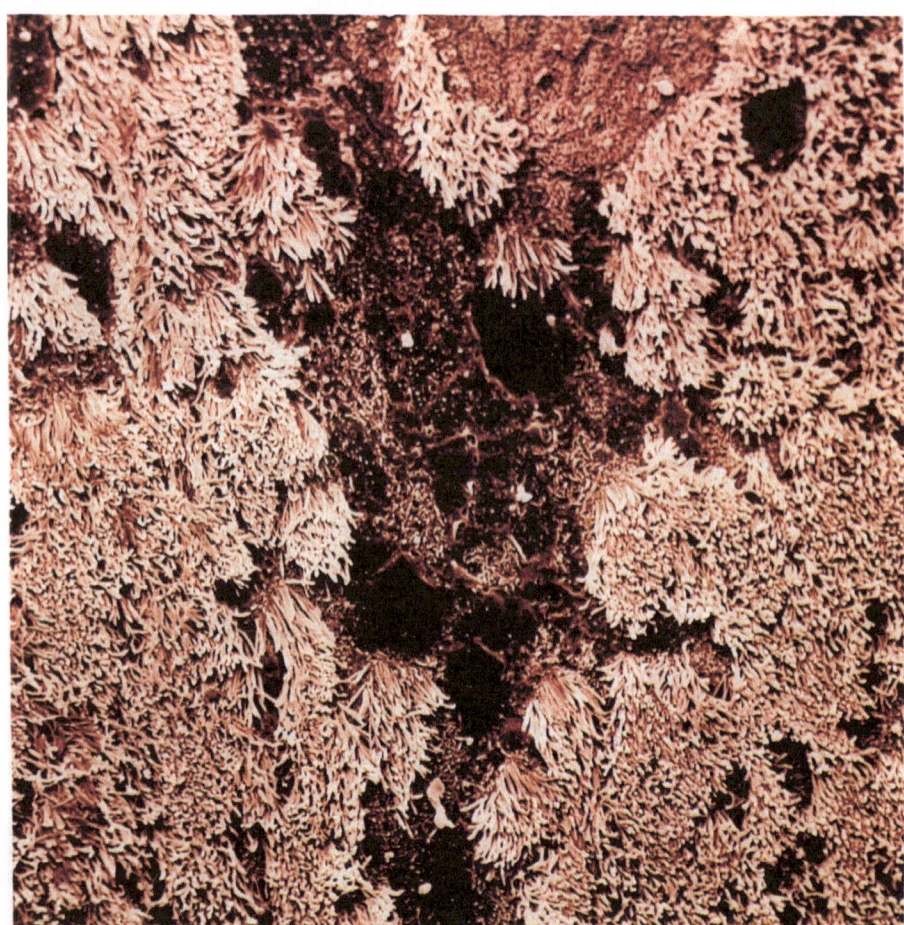

Fig. 7.3. The respiratory mucosal deciliation causes exposure of the basal cell layer (×655)

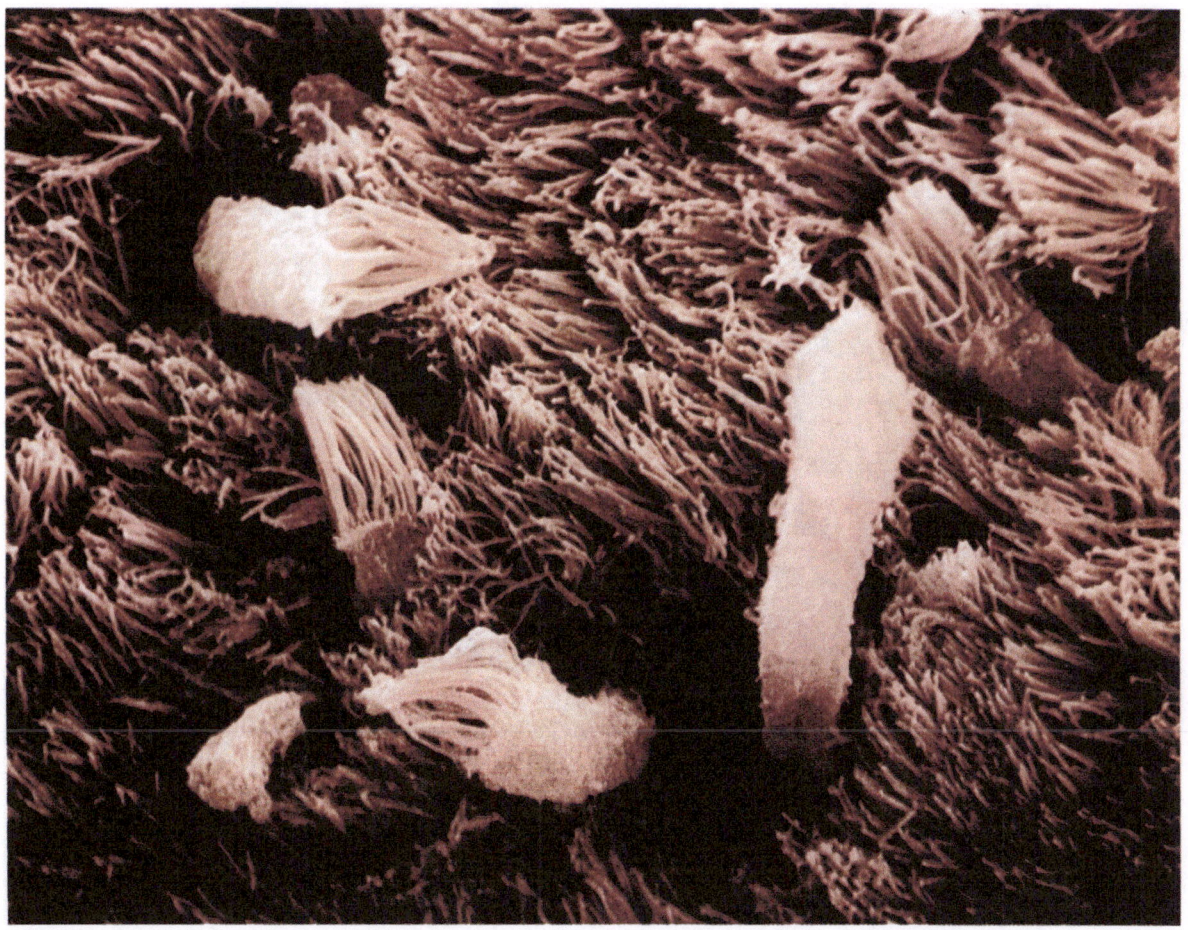

Fig. 7.4. The first visible change to the normal respiratory epithelial structure after exposure to any injury is the sloughing of the dead ciliated cells, which are more sensitive than the goblet cells because of their greater differentiation (×2100)

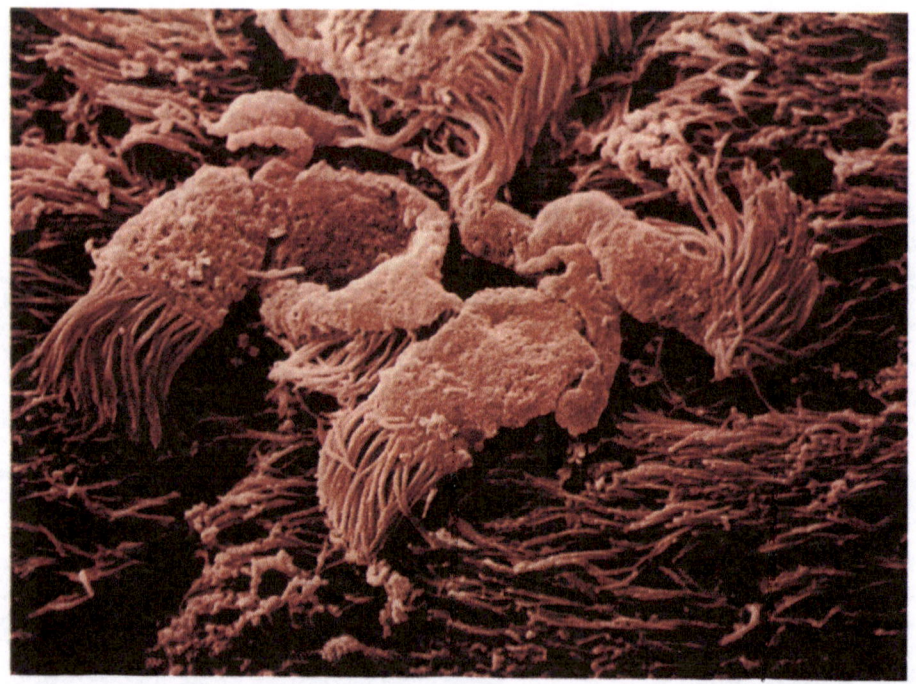

Fig. 7.5. In this micrograph many ciliated cells and cellular debris can be seen lying on the respiratory epithelium, which already shows loss of the metachronal coordination of the ciliary movement (×2620)

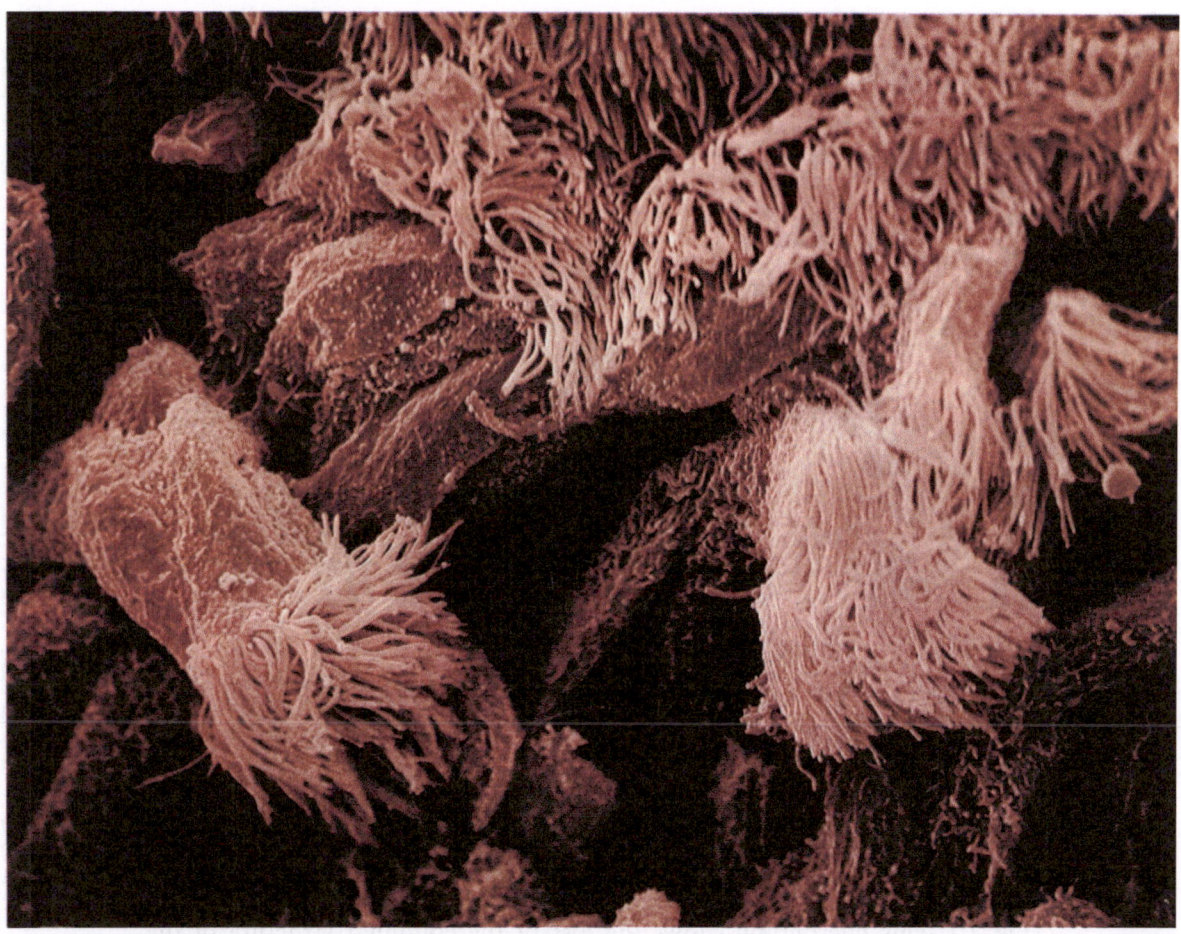

Fig. 7.6. A more advanced stage of epithelial destruction. Besides the cellular sloughing, alterations in the normal architecture of the respiratory mucosa can be seen ($\times$1850)

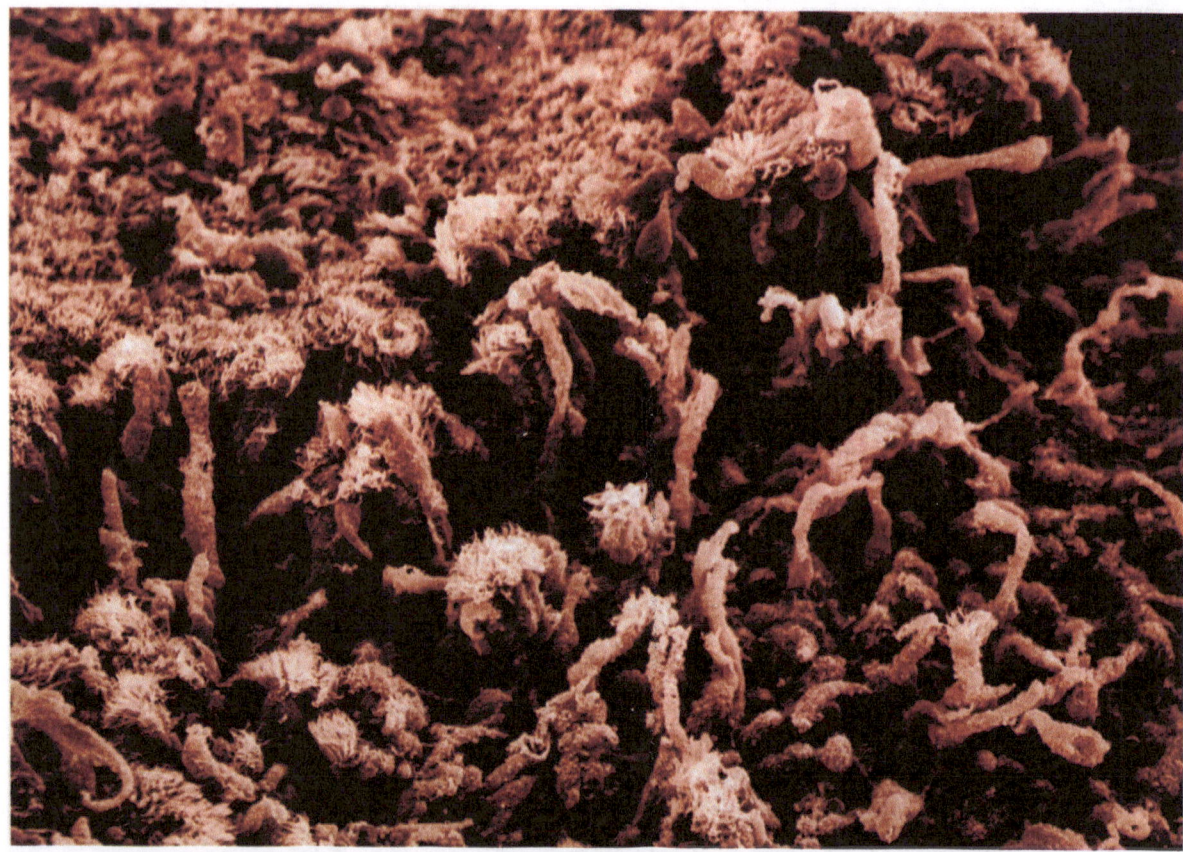

Fig. 7.7. This micrograph shows the loss of the columnar structure of the respiratory epithelium and the disorganization of the ciliated and basal cells (×850)

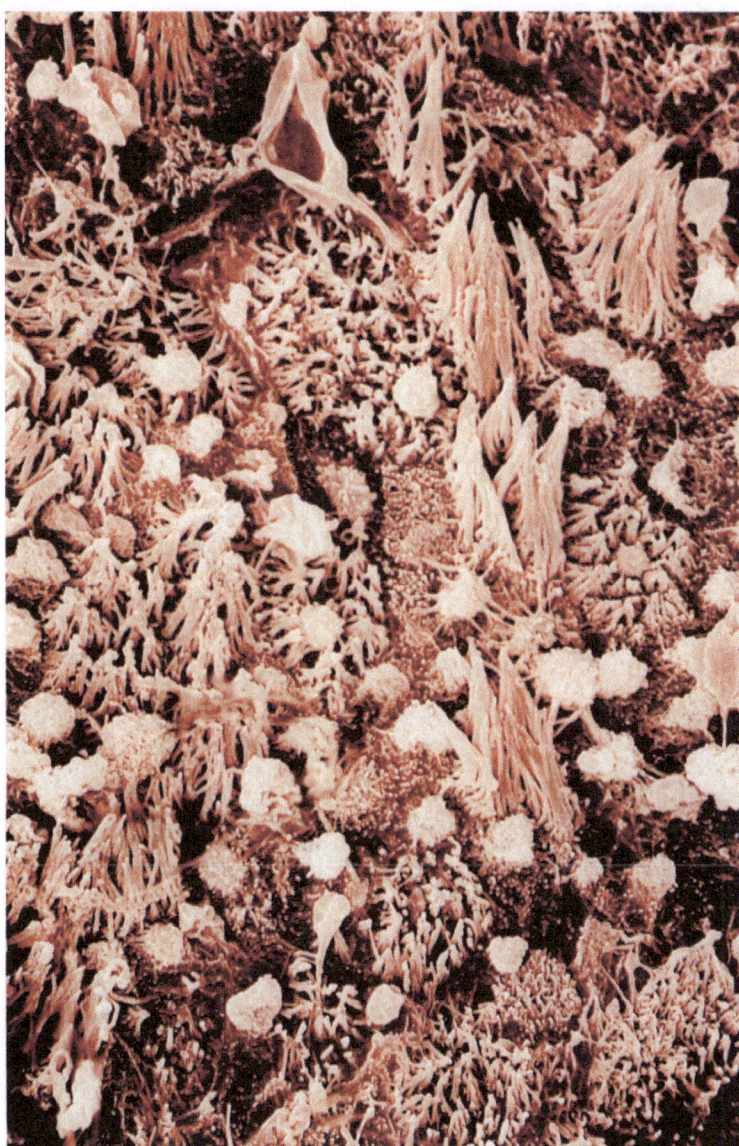

Fig. 7.8. The degree of damage progresses until more drastic changes of the morphological features of the normal respiratory mucosa can be seen: severe deciliation, grouping of the remaining cilia, and many cells with shorter young cilia, expressing an attempt of ciliary regeneration (×800)

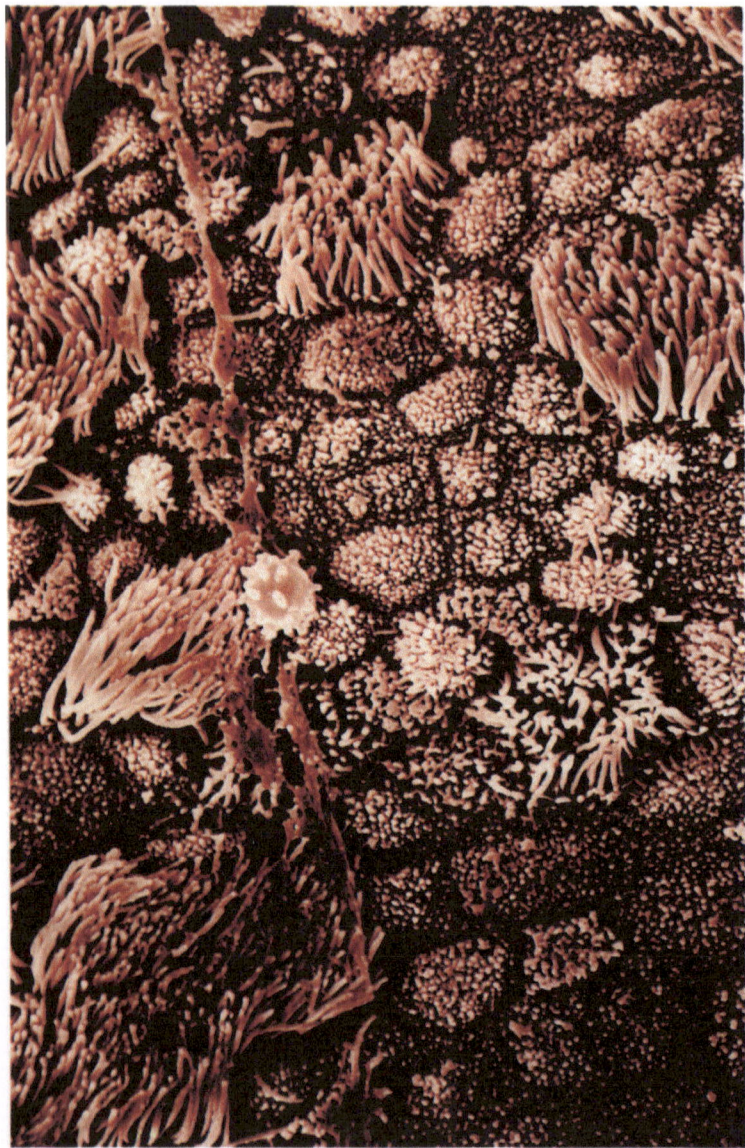

Fig. 7.9. This area of the respiratory mucosa is lined almost entirely by nonciliated cells whose surfaces are covered by small microvilli: this causes a marked impairment of the mucociliary clearance (×2400)

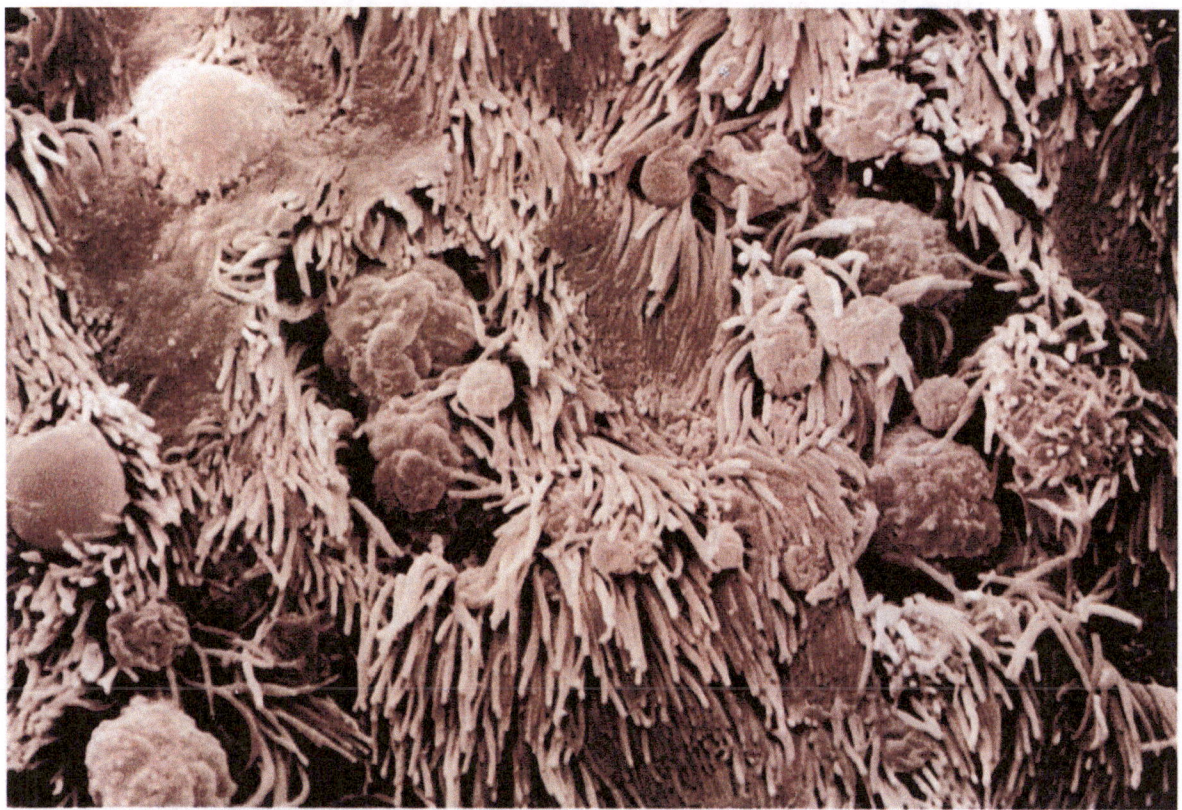

Fig. 7.10. Chronic bronchitis is characterized by a situation like that shown in this picture. The excessive production of mucus with altered physicochemical characteristics glues the cilia, which are not in a vertical position but lying flat. The goblet cells increase in volume and in number. Mucociliary clearance is impaired (×2980)

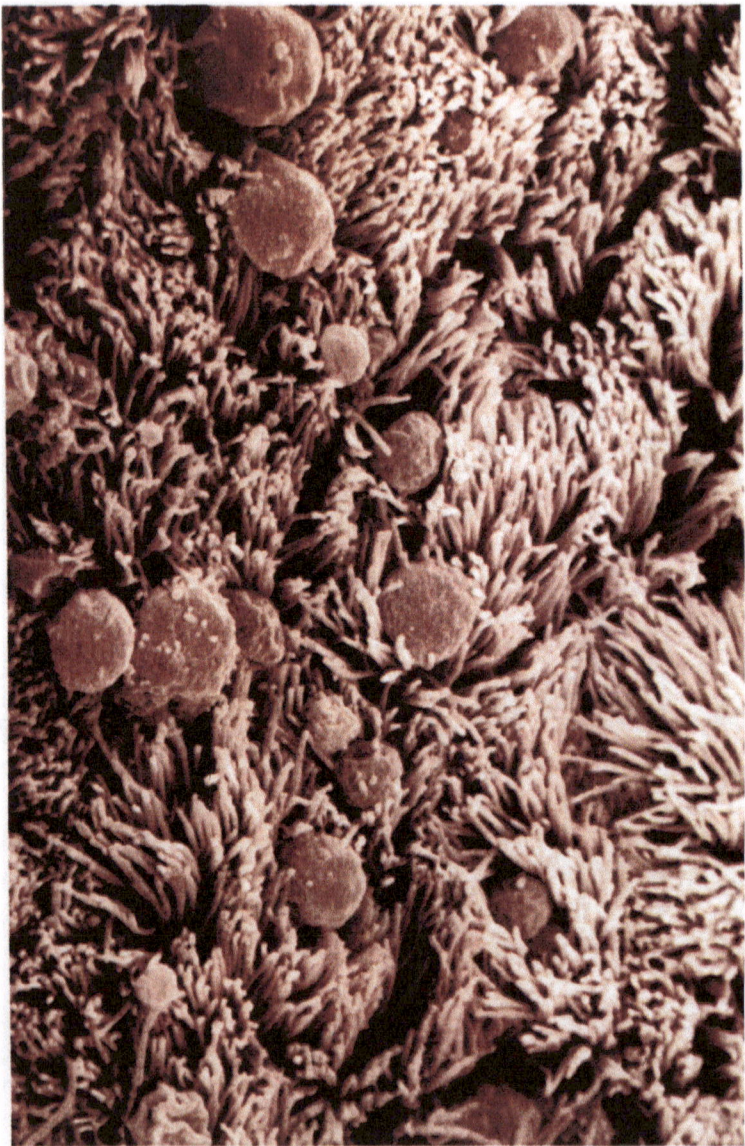

Fig. 7.11. After treatment with a mucoactive drug (SCMC-Lys), the goblet cells appear reduced in number and less swollen, the cilia are less glued each other, and mucociliary clearance should improve (×2620)

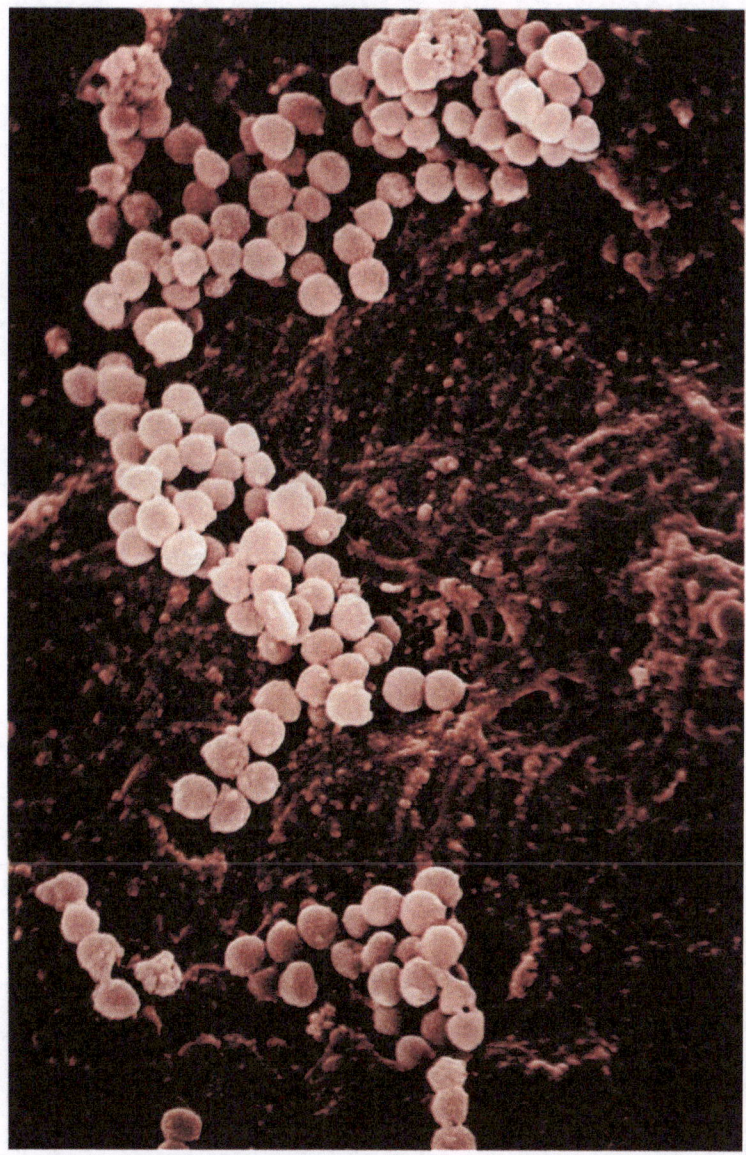

Fig. 7.12. Many bacteria (e.g., *Staphylococcus aureus*) are able to adhere to the tracheobronchial secretions, thus causing bronchopulmonary infection (×5000)

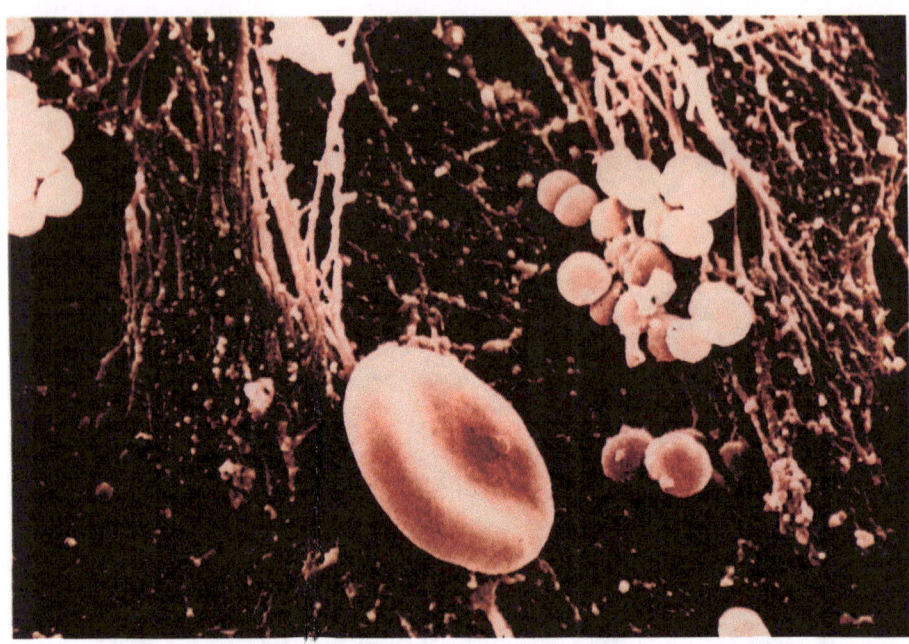

Fig. 7.13. The bacteria are trapped in the mucous filaments. Note the relative sizes of the bacterial cells and the erythrocyte (×6200)

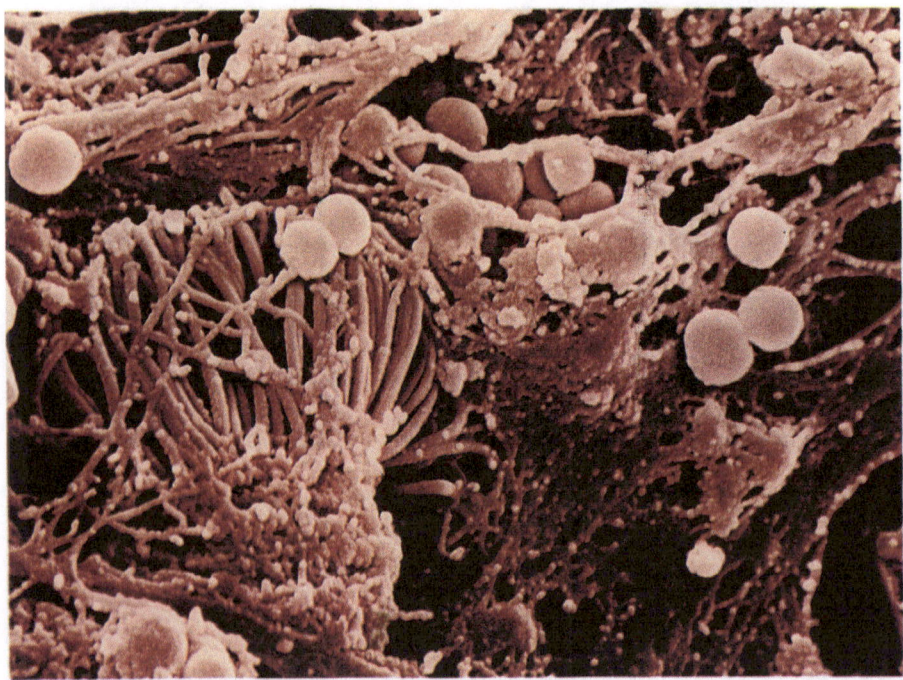

Fig. 7.14. A pathological condition characterized by a mucous layer which traps the underlying cilia, together with numerous bacteria *(S. aureus)*. The appearance is completely different from the physiological ones shown in Chaps. 2 and 3 (×7400)

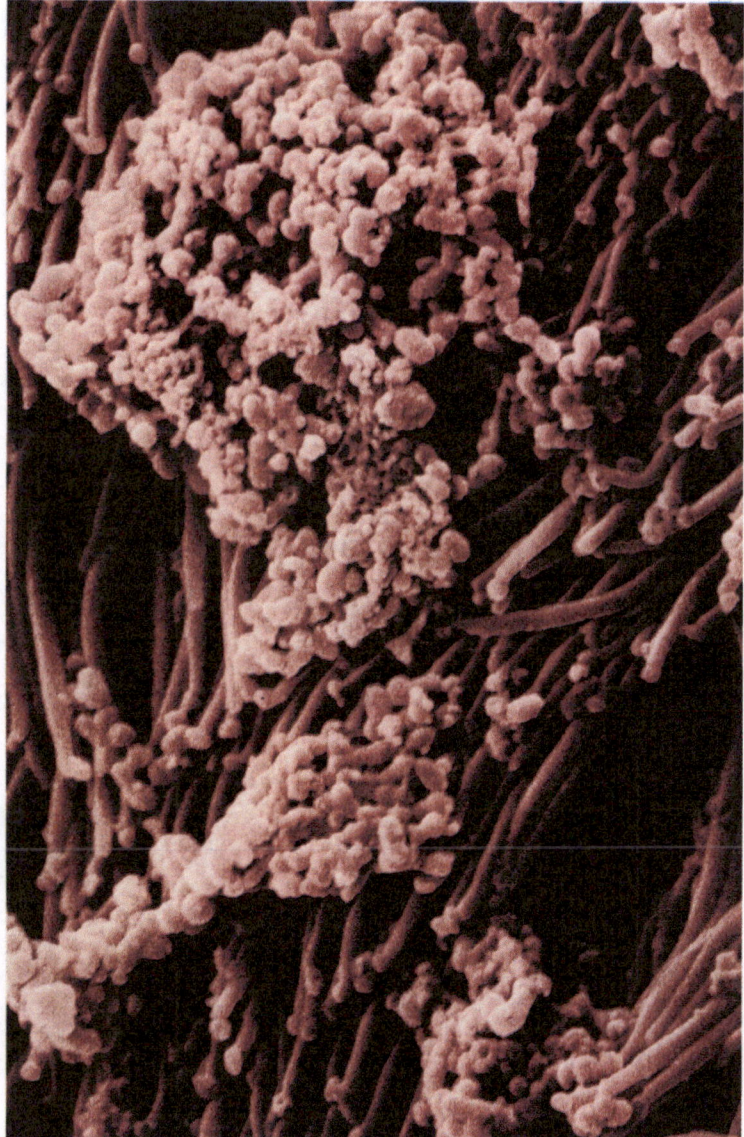

Fig. 7.15. Bacteria can also adhere directly to the cilia and their tips (×4000)

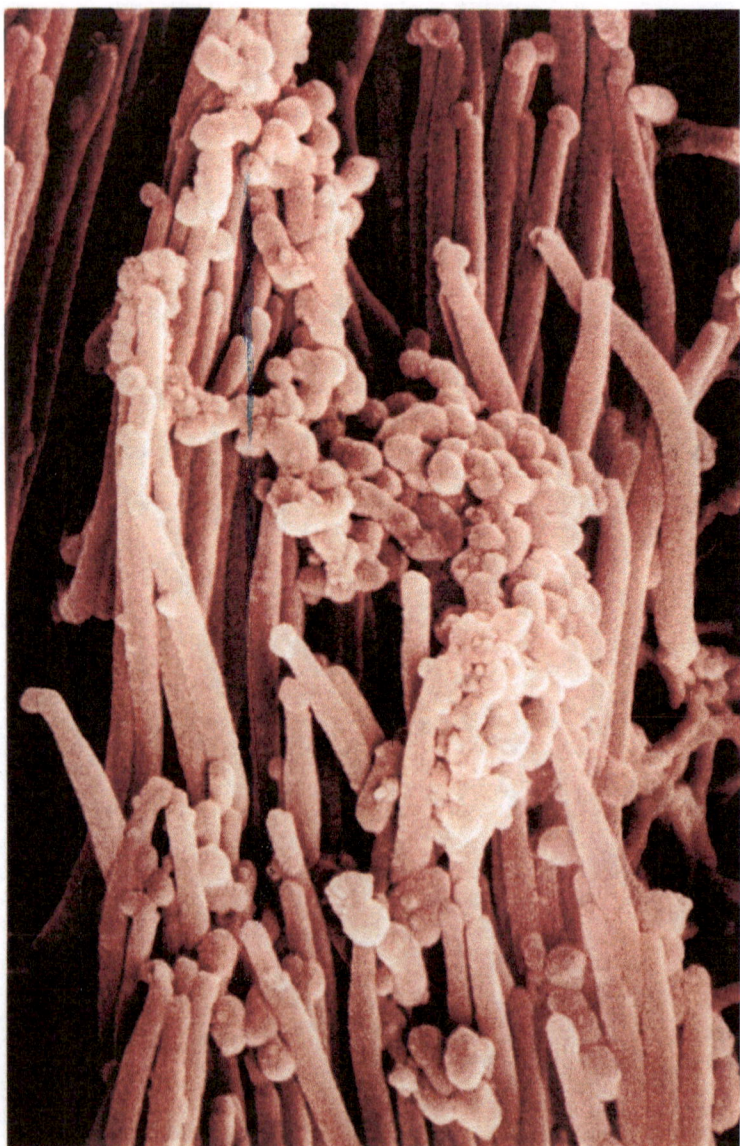

Fig. 7.16. The bacteria that adhere to the cilia of the respiratory mucosa synthesize several toxins which alter the ciliary beat (×5600)

Subject Index